whatever happened to
patient 2410

by
minda lazarov

Ideas into Books®
WESTVIEW
Kingston Springs, Tennessee

ii

Ideas into Books®
W E S T V I E W
P.O. Box 605
Kingston Springs, TN 37082
www.publishedbywestview.com

ISBN 978-1-62880-029-6

First edition, September 2014

Photo credits: Front and back cover photos by Barry Sulkin. Other photos are
from the author's personal collection.

Cover design by Shea Lazarov Sulkin.

The author gratefully acknowledges permission to reprint lyrics from
"Blessing" by Jonell Mosser, John and Johanna Hall, used by permission of
the authors.

The author gratefully acknowledges permission to reprint "Optimism" by
Jane Hirshfield, © Jane Hirshfield, from *Given Sugar, Given Salt* (NY:
HarperCollins, 2001); used by permission of Jane Hirshfield, all rights
reserved.

Digitally printed in the United States of America on acid free paper.

acknowledgements and dedication

Forty years. The span of time Moses needed to lead the Israelites out of bondage and back to their homeland.

In the forty years between the terms of Presidents Eisenhower and George W. Bush, I experienced a full body assault from several bouts of cancer and other not so benign tumors. This book is the story of that four decade struggle and the valuable knowledge I gained about getting in and out of the health care system with the best possible outcome.

I spent hundreds of hours combing through medical records, talking with family, friends and health care providers and unsticking the pages of my memory to reconstruct the events with accuracy. Yet, in some instances, I was left with only my imagination to fill in the missing details and recreate dialogue. You probably wouldn't want the final product to be any closer to reality.

Most of the names of the many doctors, nurses, and other providers are shortened beyond recognition. I've chosen to honor a handful of extraordinary practitioners to whom I owe my life by giving their full names.

To health, insurance liberty, and the pursuit of a manageable health care system, I dedicate this book.

Minda Lazarov, Patient 2410
May 12, 2010

patient 2410, minda lazarov, born 1955

1970	Neck and chest radiation for Hodgkin's lymphoma
1971	Surgery #1: Laparotomy Chemotherapy and radiation for Hodgkin's lymphoma Surgery #2: Laparotomy
1972	Surgery #3: Laparotomy
1979	Hodgkin's lymphoma recurrence with chemotherapy treatment
1992	Surgery #4: Removal of ovarian tumor (oophorectomy)
1995	Surgery #5: Right breast cancer and mastectomy
1998	Surgery #6: Left breast cancer and mastectomy Surgery #7: Reconstructive breast surgeries Surgery #8: Brain surgery for removal of acoustic neuroma
2006	Surgery #9: Brain surgery for removal of left optic nerve tumor (meningioma)
2007	Surgery #10: Removal of right jaw tumor (schwannoma)
2009	Epstein-Barr virus related B-cell Lymphoma with chemotherapy treatment

table of contents

whatever happened to
patient 2410

chapter one

2005, OCTOBER

She said yes. I said no. She said yes. I said maybe.

In more than twenty-five years of public speaking, I had seldom bared the wounds of my wrestling match with the cancer demons. An invitation to expose these vulnerabilities to two hundred breast cancer survivors and their families seemed like a stretch far beyond my area of expertise. That's why, when Lee Hederman of the American Cancer Society asked me to speak at the Reach to Recovery Fashion Show, my first response was *No.*

I had been waiting years for an invitation to model in their annual fundraiser fashion show, and if Lee had asked me that, I would have said, *You bet!* I envisioned myself swaggering down the runway with my handsomely updated, upright chest mounds on full display. I smiled to myself. *Ms. Hederman, I'm your gal! I will not disappoint you! I look best in blue!*

But instead, she asked, "Would you give the opening address?"

She caught me off guard. "You want me to do what?"

"We'd like you to speak to our volunteers and survivors about your experience with breast cancer."

Her innocent request dashed my delusion. She wanted me to pontificate rather than promenade? She must have assumed I had something noteworthy to say, but although I felt honored, I was much more interested in strutting my stuff. Then it struck me. If I spoke this year, maybe I would get my big modeling break next year.

"Well, maybe. May I think about what I might say and get back to you?" I asked.

Saying no to an organization that had probably played a significant role in my survival would clutter my mostly-clean conscience. Surely I could come up with something meaningful to say.

As soon as I hung up the phone, though, a flood of memories overwhelmed me. I've endured a lot of physical abuse over the years—surgery, surgery and more surgery, radiation, chemotherapy and more chemotherapy, intrusive tests, poking, prodding. But unlike the physical abuse of domestic violence, these experiences buoyed my soul and self-confidence. When Lee's call came, I'd reached the stage of my odyssey where the cause—staying alive—clearly had been worth the effort, with a many-fold return on the tidy sum I'd paid.

Years earlier I'd begun recording this journey and the lessons learned about finding my way through the medical system. That manuscript lay untouched and unfinished in a manila folder in a rusting four-drawer metal file cabinet in our attic next to our 1977 tax returns. Lack of stamina from my eighth major surgery and lack of confidence that I could add anything to the crowded arena of cancer survivor stories had ended my brief stint as a memoirist. In those few pages, however, were the beginnings of what I hoped could be an inspirational speech worthy of sharing with my comrades.

Two months later, I incorporated these random reflections into my opening address at the Vanderbilt Loew's Hotel in Nashville. Demetria Kalodimos, the charismatic anchorwoman of Nashville's primetime television news cast, introduced me to the attendees who were enjoying their chicken breasts. These women, and a few men, were anxiously awaiting the runway appearance of their sisters, daughters, mothers, and wives—women who had given all or part of their own breasts in exchange for life.

I began my talk against the backdrop of inattentive luncheoners focused on their thirty-dollar-a-plate of food. Within a couple of minutes, the clatter of forks and knives was replaced by silence. As I unfolded my intimate story to this crowd of strangers, the expanding volume of their silence was all I needed. Their attention let me know it was time to tell my saga about living in the inferno of a faltering human body and its would-be savior, the American health care system.

1970, FEBRUARY

Adolescence requires walking a precarious tightrope between individuality and conformity. When we're teens, if we shift too far toward expressing our individuality, we risk falling into the abyss of weirdos, forever feeling out of sync with our peers. Dip too far the other way, and we disappear into a fuzzy homogenous haze and spend the next thirty years trying to figure out who we are. No training is offered for mastering this balancing act. The door of adolescence suddenly blows open, and we're pushed through. Our mentors for maneuvering developmental changes—our parents—are no longer suitable for the job. So we're forced to go it alone. The simultaneous urge to both hold onto and let go of the parental tether is the first of many paradoxes muddling the adolescent years.

Most of us burst through the entry and quickly mutate into the two-faced monster we euphemistically call a teenager. There is the eager-beaver side—energetic, naïvely hopeful, and open to new ideas. The flip side is the sloth—always in need of sleep at the wrong time, grumpy, cynical, and depressingly narrow-minded. When the two sides collide, run as fast as you can. It's not a pretty sight.

When I was fourteen, with budding breasts competing with a burgeoning nose for dominance over my self-esteem, I was beginning to feel the daily struggle between the two faces of Minda. Yet, miraculously, the two sides merged over the next year and have since never parted, forming an armor stronger than the titanium plates now holding my skull together. The first step toward that union began in an unlikely venue, a junior high school gym class in my hometown of Memphis, Tennessee.

The yellowed oak gym floor of Richland Junior High School was always spotless and shiny with a buffed coat of lacquer. Daily workouts under the command of our gym teacher, Miss Winstead, were mandatory. On this early spring day, the directive for the hour was to stand in line until we reached the front, then charge three steps forward and toss the brown leather ball into the basket. I stood in line with eight of my peers. We were all dressed out in matching wrinkled white gym suits awaiting Miss Winstead's shrill whistle to get the line moving. It was hard to say which we disliked more, Miss Winstead or our gym suits. Surely a man designed the embarrassingly ugly attire gathered at the waist and abruptly ending at mid thigh.

I held my place in line, dreading my turn to make the toss. One minute I was worried about whether I could pull off a display of athletic talent that would make up for my ridiculous duds. The next minute, the room was spinning. I felt I was on a Tilt-a-Whirl at the state fair, spiraling faster and faster out of control.

As quickly as it started, it was over. I looked around. No one seemed to notice. The secret of my momentary loss of control was mine alone. I took my place at the front of the line, but as the ball flew through the air, a voice was yelling at me: *Something is wrong.*

A few days later in geometry class, a fleeting physiological misstep jolted me again. Mrs. Newsom was droning about the Pythagorean theorem when, all of a sudden, I lost my breath, as if I had just been socked in the stomach. Struggling to inhale and catch a breath, I raised my hand, stumbled to the front of the room, and whispered to Mrs. Newsom, "May I go home? I feel really weird. I can't breathe."

Mrs. Newsom sent me to the principal's office where I signed out. In the orderly middle-class milieu of the South in 1970, naïve trust in young teens still prevailed, and a verbal complaint of illness was the only ticket I needed to enter the world beyond the school grounds. As I left through the red double front doors and walked a few blocks home, my feet felt like lead, and my lungs felt squeezed. I could inhale only a brief gasp of air.

The wind was blowing hard, and the narrow sidewalk seemed to be taking me to some frightening destination. I wanted to turn back, stop the clock. I longed for the safety of home. As I pushed forward with a labored series of puffs, I noted familiar surroundings. For an instant, the pink Mary Kay Cadillac parked in the Kopacek driveway diverted my attention. How many times had I walked down this sidewalk without a care in the world? *I want to be home. Mom, Dad, where are you? What's wrong with my lungs? I can't breathe!*

By the time I got home, my lungs had snapped back into action, inflating and deflating as lungs are supposed to do. I entered the kitchen door. Dad was sitting at the table reading the newspaper. Israel Lazarov, or Laz as most people called him, was forty-eight at the time. This was Tuesday, his day off from the neighborhood grocery store across town that he co-owned with my uncle. I joined him at the table.

"You're home early. What's wrong?" Dad asked rather casually, as opposed to freaked out as my mother would have been.

"I was having this weird problem breathing, so they let me come home. I feel fine now, though."

I played it down, convincing my father and myself I had experienced a passing abnormality that meant no harm. But convincing my mother was another story. She insisted on taking me to the pediatrician. Dr. A. saw nothing out of the ordinary on the X-ray.

A few weeks later, the breathing difficulty returned with a severe cough, a high fever, and a swollen lip and eyelids. Dr. A. labeled the condition an allergy and sent us home. As the fever persisted and the lethargy worsened, he tested me for rheumatic fever. The test was negative. With no more tricks to pull out of his doctor's bag, he conjured up a diagnosis of streptococcus and prescribed penicillin. All the symptoms eventually disappeared.

Months went by with no more physical peculiarities. During the summer, I accompanied my mother to a public health screening for tuberculosis. This debilitating, highly infectious disease of the lungs had affected almost one million Americans during the height of its fury in the 1950s and 1960s. A killer since the reign of the Egyptian pharaohs, TB was on the decline, but still dreaded. National efforts were launched to further curb its spread. Fortunately, a quick, inexpensive radiogram (chest X-ray) easily identified carriers of the disease. Mobile screening trailers travelled across the United States testing health care workers, teachers, and others in contact with the public, even grocery store clerks. By requiring these X-rays, the federal government was able to cut off the major pathways of TB transmission.

My mother, Matilda Saperstein Lazarov, who was a fifth grade teacher at the time, dragged me along for the required look and see of her lungs. The screening trailer was nothing fancy. Today, most of us wouldn't trust health care dispensed from such a modest, rundown facility.

As my mother signed in with the technician at the entrance, she asked, "Can my daughter get an X-ray, too?"

This was long before the days of the cost-conscious health care industry, so the man in white replied in the manner any gracious southerner would. "Sure, honey. Step right up."

A few days later, a short but ominous letter arrived in our mailbox.

> *Dear Mrs. Lazarov: Your X-ray is negative, but your daughter's X-ray revealed a possible heart condition. We recommend you take her to a doctor for follow-up.*

My mother wasted no time scheduling an appointment with the pediatrician.

"Nothing to be alarmed about," Dr. A. reassured my mother. "Minda is just standing in an awkward position, producing shadows on the X-ray. She's fine."

A mother's intuition, that shadowy, witchlike skill that spontaneously appears at the birth of a child, saved my life. Mothers watch. Mothers worry. Mothers deduce. My mother's intuition was just beginning round one of this fight. As she observed my Twiggy-thin adolescent body dragging along on its march toward maturity, she questioned the physician's wisdom. Yet who did she think she was to second-guess a medical doctor? In 1970 we still resided under the all-knowing reign of Doctors Know Best.

Mom's maternal itch persisted over the summer and into the school year. Like the phantom cop who always seems to be tailing when you're speeding, her maternal voice of worry could not be subdued. Each day I came home from school and plopped down on the white Naugahyde sofa in front of the reruns of *Gilligan's Island*. Listless and lacking stamina for extracurricular activities, I watched the wacky adventures of Gilligan, the Professor, Mary Ann, and "the rest," day after day.

Most days I drifted off to the sounds of the skipper harassing Gilligan as he fumbled yet another task.

Something is wrong, thought my mother. Time for a second opinion. She turned to the trusted family GP. Examination number two by the crusty old practitioner who should have long since retired revealed nothing. Same conclusion, different reasons.

"She's just a nervous child. That's why she's so thin. And X-rays can be deceiving. Stop worrying about her." His opinions emerged perhaps from career fatigue rather than scientific logic.

The relentless nagging of Mother Matilda's intuition drove us to a third opinion. A well-known cardiologist with a spotless reputation stepped into the ring for round three. On the Friday after Thanksgiving, Mom hit pay dirt—or in this case you might call it a pool of quicksand. Dr. Salky took one look at the X-ray, another look at my five-foot-five, ninety-pound wisp-of-a-woman frame, listened to the heartfelt woes of a mother tracking the scent of trouble, and palpated a lump in my neck. Duh. *Something's wrong.*

But he was cool, with no alarming tone in his voice. "There's something not right with Minda's X-ray. And I feel a swollen lymph node in her neck. I'd like to admit her to Baptist Hospital on Tuesday and have it removed, so we can know precisely what we're dealing with."

The surgery was uneventful. The diagnosis was not. Six days after the office visit to Dr. Salky, a somber-looking troop marched into my hospital room and lined up at the end of my bed. Dr. Salky, along with the surgeon, my mother, and my father stood at attention as the sentence was pronounced.

"You have Hodgkin's disease, a disease of the lymph nodes," Dr. Salky said. "We've told your parents we're very hopeful. You are young, female, and in good health. The outlook is good."

The C word was never spoken. My forever upbeat father looked tired and distraught. He usually showed no visible signs of fluctuations in physical or emotional status unless he felt unbearable pain. When the hurt was too severe, his eyes showed the truth.

On the other hand, I always knew where my mother stood. She was crying.

I felt confused. I thought, *They're overreacting. Parents are so weird.*

Little did I realize the first blow had been struck by a knife that would whittle away at my body, part by part, for decades to come. At that moment, however, I had a naïve teenage brain on my side. This chameleon-like organ can morph into a protective armor at crucial times. A skepticism of the authority of elders—people over twenty—can combine with an uncanny ability to place a positive spin on factoids. In my case, this adolescent high-and-mightiness served me well. I'd never known anyone with a serious illness. I hadn't heard anything but good news. They removed a small lump from my neck. It was gone. They had a diagnosis. They know what to do. *So let's get on with it.*

The next day, they got on with it. There was no time to lose. The radiation treatments began. I was wheeled through the hospital to a cavernous room for the first of my daily treatments. Smack dab in the middle of the room was a lone stainless steel examining table with a walrus-sized piece of heavy metal and enamel-encased equipment hovering in the air above the table. The table and the hanging legless walrus were surrounded by empty space—lots of it. There was room enough for ten couples to take their places for ballroom dancing. As I moved from my wheelchair onto the table, I was given a very brief description of what was to come.

"I need you to lie very still on your back while I make some lines on you to direct the radiation to the right place," the technician said. No "how do you do" or "this will not hurt."

I stretched out on my back, feeling a sense of urgency to follow his instructions. What came next seemed like an elementary drawing lesson to help a four-year-old stay inside the lines.

The technician drew several thick lines on my neck and chest with a chestnut-brown marker. The lines formed a long inch-wide rectangle extending the length of my neck. Another set of lines formed an odd-shaped border around my breasts, kind of like a graph of the peaks and valleys of the Dow Jones Average. It's interesting I have no recollection of the shock of baring my chest to this stranger, but I can remember how many couples would fit in the room.

Next, he pulled the limbless walrus down closer to my neck and chest. It hung in a parallel position to my recumbent body, about a foot directly above me. A small window shade magically opened up in the belly of the walrus, revealing a clear glass window to its insides. A light was emitted through this window and projected onto my chest. The technician worked for several minutes to get the walrus's light to completely fill in the polygon without crossing outside the lines. When the technician was sufficiently pleased with the illuminated area, he rolled a sheet of clear glass into place between me and the walrus's belly.

Here's where twentieth century, state-of-the-art medical science relied on the Hasbro Toy Company for high-tech design principles. The technician rolled up a table of building blocks next to me and the walrus. His goal was downright simple, yet laden with dangerous implications. Using the light as a guide, he formed a perfect border of blocks to contain the cobalt radiation beams within the lines. Misplacement of the blocks would result in scattered rays that could miss their mark. And a poor marksman could mean more cancer down the road.

With a focus similar to a preschooler struggling to arrange the blocks in a way to make his mother proud, the walrus technician intently placed the first block on the glass tray. He adjusted the block, moving it just a tiny bit to the left. He adjusted the block once again, satisfied that it perfectly aligned with the border he'd drawn. The technician repeated the pattern with the other blocks until he completed the masterpiece he had envisioned. *Finis!*

He flipped a switch. The light from the walrus's belly went dark and the window shade closed.

The final step spooked the hell out of me.

"I need you to lie very, very still. Do not move any part of your body. It won't take long—just a few minutes." The technician failed to explain what "it" was.

He walked out of the room. As he shut the door behind him, I heard the heavy thud of a massive bank vault door. It *was* a massive vaulted door, designed to protect the innocent observer from unwanted radiation. In this case, I was not the innocent. Alone in the vacuous tomb with the walrus looming over me, I thought, *What have I gotten myself into?*

The window in the belly opened once again. This time a long buzz blurted out from deep within the walrus's innards. Five minutes later, the walrus ceased his mournful song. The belly window closed, and all was quiet. I didn't feel a thing.

The vault door opened, and the now cheerful technician entered with a big smile on his face. "We're done!"

He swept the blocks away. "You can go back to your room now." Mr. Congeniality made no effort to lessen my anxiety or answer any burning questions. He assisted me into the wheelchair and rolled me away.

The next day I received radiation treatment number two. Same time. Same routine.

After four days of outings to the vaulted dance hall with the walrus and Mr. Congeniality, I received a call from one of my best friends. I had been in the hospital for more than a week and had not seen or heard from a single friend. Hospital policy dictated that youngsters, including teens, were unwelcome visitors, apparently obstructive to the healing process. My mother adhered to the dictate, prohibiting calls to allow for rest.

I was sitting up in the hospital bed staring off into space when the bedside phone rang.

"How's it going?" my friend said.

I have no recollection of the tenor of my friend's voice. I just remember the conversation, a conversation I will never forget.

"I'm okay. Feeling pretty good actually," I replied.

The caller explained that several of our friends from the Jewish youth group, Levy AZA, were at an old warehouse cleaning out storage space for Le Bonheur Children's Hospital.

"We found this set of *Funk and Wagnalls Encyclopedia* and looked up Hodgkin's disease. Did you know you have cancer? And it says here it's fatal. You may not have long to live."

No male or female pitch is attached to the memory of the caller. Only the message remains on file. I had cancer.

I had two very valuable filters processing the news for me, my genes and my arrogant teenage psyche. As I was to experience again and again, I had inherited a gene from my father allowing me to hear the news, register the shock, ponder its meaning, and accept that which I could not control. The Be Here Now gene. Some of us have it; some of us don't. I didn't study ten years under a guru to connect with this wisdom. I just won the gene lottery and inherited it.

News of an alleged prognosis that could have shattered my youthful dreams quickly ricocheted off my internal armor. At fifteen, I moved through the stages of anger, confusion, blame, and recovery in less than the time it took for my now faceless friend to share the blunt tidings. (These days it takes longer.)

The catalyst for the lightning speed of my rebound was my teenage confidence in a personal storehouse of bogus knowledge. My immature intellect led me to a fast conclusion. *Hogwash! I feel fine. I am fine. We have a bump in the road here, but my bodily unit is going to glide over the bump intact.*

A few good friends who were at the warehouse later reflected on the episode.

Jeff said, "We really didn't know what was wrong with you other than you had this strange diagnosis of Hodgkin's disease that none of us had ever heard of."

Carol, one of my best friends, said, "One day you were there, and the next day you dropped off the face of the earth. We weren't allowed to see you."

Unbeknownst to me, rumors had been flying. There was a shroud of mystery around my disappearance and diagnosis. Jeff had scoured the dusty 1955 edition of *Funk and Wagnalls*. Volume *H* was one of the remaining volumes still in the box they'd found, and as Jeff read the fifteen-year-old description aloud, Carol took the news hard, wailing on his shoulder for the next thirty minutes. Serious illness, death, and dying were alien to all of us.

When the gang regained their composure, someone suggested, "Let's get down to the bottom of this and call Minda."

Many years later, when I was exploring memories with Carol in preparation for writing this book, she apologized profusely for the lapse in group judgment to call me. I harbored no hard feelings. At fifteen, I was unfazed by the news. I was simply grateful to reconnect with friends.

The litany of procedures up to that point in my hospital stay was minor—an X-ray, some blood work, one small incision in my neck to remove a swollen lymph node, and the seemingly harmless radiation treatments. None of these procedures caused physical pain. The next procedure, however, led me to a doctor whose techniques were reminiscent of Dr. Farb, the sadistic dentist in *Little Shop of Horrors*.

Our initial introduction was misleading. Disguised as another chipper medical do-gooder performing another simple procedure, he had the task of obtaining a sample of marrow from the inside of my pelvis. When I think back on this first bone marrow biopsy, the thorny memories mesh into a Wild West scene. Someone's amputating my leg with a saw, grinding through the bone while I'm biting on a bullet.

In actuality the doctor did not use a saw. He inserted a hefty needle through my lower back into my pelvis bone, drilling into the soupy center. Here, inside the glutinous marrow, resided white blood cells whose destination might ultimately be one of my lymph nodes. These cells could provide additional clues about the origin and extent of the cancer.

The results came back the next day. Positive—the cancer had made its way to the marrow. However, a second doctor interpreted the results as negative for evidence of disease—no signs of cancer in the marrow. Dr. Salky must have asked himself, *Where do we go from here?*

Elaborate flow charts based on test results often serve as road maps to help direct physicians to a specific route of treatment, but inconclusive results lead to fuzzy directions. When there are no clear road signs, physicians rely on experience in navigating the maze. Wisely, Dr. Salky referred me and my family to St. Jude Children's Research Hospital, fortuitously located in our hometown of Memphis. Even back then, it was an internationally recognized facility for the treatment of childhood cancers. Dr. Salky knew St. Jude offered the greatest likelihood for my survival.

Eleven days after I was admitted to Baptist Hospital, Mom escorted me to St. Jude, both the most comforting and the scariest place a teenage cancer kid could land.

chapter two

1970, December

On December 14, 1970, I became the two-thousand-four-hundred-and-tenth patient admitted to St. Jude Children's Research Hospital. 2410. This number is branded into every nook and cranny of my shrinking memory bank.

Bestowal of your patient number is one of the first rites of passage into the privileged membership of St. Jude alumni. Attempts to categorize people as numbers usually irritate our delicate egos. We feel our individuality is being sabotaged. However, the number 2410 renders remarkable definition to my individuality, a definition on which I have thrived for decades. It is my badge of honor.

2410.2410. 2410.

It echoes in my mind like the winning number of a raffle that's called out again and again until the winner steps forward. It makes me want to run to the front of the room where the prize ticket is being waved in the air. *2410. That's me! I won! I'm a St. Jude survivor!* I beam inside and out when I reveal my membership in this elite group.

Founded in 1962 by the actor and comedian Danny Thomas, the hospital had almost a decade of experience in treating childhood cancers by the time I was admitted. The passion of a promise made by Mr. Thomas to the patron saint of hopeless causes, St. Jude Thaddeus, is legendary in the halls of the hospital. It underlies the zeal of the entire St. Jude staff.

Danny Thomas was a young man when he pleaded to St. Jude for a purpose and direction to his life. Years as an entertainer led to just moderate success, then a lull—the smashing breakthrough never arrived. With a growing family, Danny was struggling to stay balanced on an economic and emotional tight-wire. His prayer to St. Jude "to help me find my way in life" gave birth to a grounding vision. His promise to build a shrine to honor St. Jude eventually evolved into a mission to establish a hospital for needy children.

When his career finally took off with his stand-up comedy, movie roles, and the popular sitcom *Make Room for Daddy*, he made good on his promise. A Catholic priest and native Tennessean urged Danny to build the hospital in Memphis. As the former bishop of his family church in Toledo where Danny had been confirmed, Cardinal Stritch persuaded Danny to locate the hospital in this southern city where the need was great and in close proximity to a medical center, roads and public transportation.

Danny and his wife, Rose Marie, dedicated nearly fifty years to raising money to build and sustain the children's hospital. The facility was to be one of a kind, not only treating catastrophic childhood illnesses such as leukemia and Hodgkin's disease, but also pursuing cutting-edge research for advancing the treatment of these "hopeless causes." No one would be turned away for lack of insurance or ability to pay. Regardless of race, religion, ethnicity, or financial resources, all patients and their families would be treated equally.

St. Jude Thaddeus must wield enormous influence. By 2011, the hospital had admitted more than twenty-nine thousand patients. The original modest facility, with a staff of one hundred twenty-five people, has mushroomed into a campus of over twenty buildings on sixty-three acres and more than three thousand employees. Children from all fifty states and more than seventy foreign countries have been treated at St. Jude. Dozens of studies are under way to identify the most effective treatment for children with a variety of life-threatening diseases, including childhood cancers, AIDS, sickle cell anemia, and genetic disorders.

Survival rates have improved dramatically since Mr. and Mrs. Thomas first opened the doors of St. Jude. Since its founding in 1962, five-year survival rates for acute lymphoblastic leukemia have risen from four percent to ninety-four percent, and for Hodgkin's disease, the rate has risen from fifty percent to ninety percent, based on national ten-year averages.

Danny and Rose Marie died in 1991 and 2000, respectively, but Danny's dream is flourishing more than ever. Both are buried on the St. Jude grounds. The torch has been passed to their children Marlo, Terre, and Tony. There is no end in sight as the treatments and body of knowledge from St. Jude continue to open doors of hope and life for the victims of catastrophic childhood disease.

Fate often gives us a sneak preview of a life-altering event that's about to be thrown in our path. I

had my first encounter with St. Jude several months
before I was diagnosed, when I toured the hospital with
my youth group sisters from Brenner BBG (B'nai Brith
Girls). I have one brief memory of the tour. The
memory plays back in one speed only—*very* slow
motion. I am pushing the front door of St. Jude open
with my hand flattened at that awkward ninety-degree
angle against the glass. My head slowly turns right, as I
look over my shoulder and smile to acknowledge
something the person behind me said. I have no
memory of a face, what she said, or what I felt after I
passed through the entrance. Only one single moment,
one single activity, representing a blind entrance into a
world unknown, but soon to be revealed on intensely
intimate terms.

From here, the images of my St. Jude past slide into
shaky territory. As I sit at my computer beginning this
chapter, instinct tells me that bringing shape to an old
trunk full of fading memories stashed away for three
decades is going to be a gut-wrenching task. My cancer
psyche—that perpetually fragile view of my physical
state of being—was birthed at St. Jude.

My fingers are on the keyboard. My heart is
palpitating. Each breath is getting heavier and shorter
as fear of the past erupts. My heart and lungs are telling
me to beware of Pandora's Box, but I'm skeptical of the
warning. Many cancer patients have endured far more
devastating experiences than I. And though I'm diving
headfirst into a deep pit of prickly memories, my hunch
is these forgotten relics have improved with age. Much
like ugly old furniture reappears years later as fine
antiques, my recollections have long awaited the light
of day to reveal their true value. So here we go.

December 15, 1970. I'm lying on my belly on an examining table. Scared shitless. Relaxing is beyond reach. It's time for another bone marrow sample. I can't stop my teeth from chattering.

I tell the nurse, "Not again. Please don't make me do this again. Can't we do this another day?"

I beg. The memory of searing pain from the "bone saw" the previous week won't go away. But the nurse is tough. Bone marrow biopsy number two must be done now. As she gives me a shot of Demerol to calm me down, my muscles begin to relax, my shoulders fall forward, my jaws unclench, my eyelids droop, and – poof – the saw is gone! I feel good. Aaahhh, the power of drugs. In no time, it's over.

This initiation into my new foster home had come after hours of questions. The previous day, we had driven from Baptist Hospital to St. Jude, no stops along the way. My devoted attendant, my mother, and I had revealed to Dr. R. the minute details of my whereabouts since birth. Dr. R. and the rest of the St. Jude staff approached each interview, each procedure, with a level of compassion and calm that clearly conveyed confidence and hope.

After the bone marrow biopsy, my mother and I were told we could go home to await the results that would determine the timing and scope of the next step. We were discharged into the land of the free!

From the time I was admitted to Baptist two weeks earlier, adults had been with me around the clock. Although they surrounded me with love and faith that all was right with the world, I longed for contact with friends, any friend. After I enjoyed a good night's rest in my own bed, Mom agreed to take me by my school following the next day's radiation treatment.

Leaving the clinic at Baptist Hospital where I was still completing the first round of radiation therapy, I felt a sense of urgency.

"Hurry, Mom, hurry! The bell for lunch rings in just fifteen minutes!"

I could not get to the car fast enough. Mom trailed behind me as I jogged through the parking lot to our baby blue Ford LTD. Mom had stayed by my side every step of the way, and I knew she would help me accomplish my next mission, reentering the world of normalcy surrounded by friends, laughter, lightness. We drove east down Poplar Avenue.

"If you hurry, I can catch up with everyone in the cafeteria. Please hurry, Mom!" The surgery and treatment had not yet dented my abundance of pubescent energy.

She turned left onto Perkins and pulled up to the curb in front of White Station School where I had begun high school as a tenth grader a few months earlier. Teenagers of all shapes and sizes were streaming through the walkway connecting the main building with the cafeteria. I hesitated to leave the car. I needed a few moments to subdue my self-consciousness as I observed the pulsating teen scene. Nervously I waited to spot a familiar face so I could slither into the crowd unnoticed by the popular Intimidators.

I saw Sharon first. I turned to Mom. "Bye. I'll see you later."

Then I flung the car door open and ran across the lawn toward the crowd, surprising myself as I called out, "Sharon, Carol, Theresa, Marcia—hey, it's me!"

Dozens of hungry teenagers stampeding toward the cafeteria doors paused and turned to look my way. The sea of bodies parted as my friends quickly surrounded me with a group hug. One day, I was gone, and then sixteen days later, I reappeared. Seemingly overnight, I was transformed into a celebrity of sorts. Everyone was excited to see me. Even Jeri, Debbie, and other popular kids took notice, kids who had failed to make eye contact with me when I passed them in the hall just two weeks earlier. While I was away, I had become a headliner in the stream of gossip among the students and teachers.

After the many embraces, the questions came flying at me: "How are you? We've been so worried! Oooohhh. What are those marks on your neck?"

Removed from the sheltered medical setting, I had totally forgotten the brownish-red brands crawling out of my collar and up my neck. The dramatic tattoos that could have made me feel freakish gave me an air of mystery, further elevating my star power. During my adolescent years, I had excelled only in academics and sewing, neither of which garnered much attention from my peers. For the first time since entering the turbulent adolescent waters, I felt strangely comfortable in my skin. Cancer was becoming a comrade in the struggle to define my persona.

1971, JANUARY

For the next four weeks, Mom and I made the trip downtown each morning for the radiation treatments. Afterward, she dropped me off at school for late morning and afternoon classes. I did not miss one treatment. Nothing, not even snow, was going to stop my mother from delivering me to the hospital for my dates with the walrus.

Meanwhile, Dad was holding down the fort, running his grocery store in south Memphis, so he was much less involved in my day-to-day care. His devotion was unequivocal, though, as were the love and support of my older sister, Reva, her husband, Mickey, and Aunt Bernice. There was never a shortage of love from my nuclear unit.

For the most part, the treatments proceeded smoothly with the exception of the periodic reappearance of an already consumed meal. To counteract the nausea, I was allowed to sit in class with one of those slender ten-ounce bottles of Coca-Cola. Vending machines, with the wide variety of enticing sugary snacks and beverages so kindly offered by the food industry today, had not yet infiltrated the school systems, so I had special permission to slip inside the secretive compound of the teachers' lounge to cop a Coke. Sitting at my desk in Algebra II class with a Coke in hand added splashes of hot pink to my smart reputation, raising the bar on the "cool" meter several notches.

My return to school was brief. The results from the latest bone marrow test along with X-rays and a dye study of lymph fluid indicated the cancerous cells had not yet traveled beyond my neck and chest. With these tests and the first round of radiation treatments behind me, it was time for the final phase of staging the lymphoma—exploratory abdominal surgery, known as a laparotomy. It was to be the first of ten major surgeries over the next thirty-six years.

Nestled in my girth were several vital organs—the spleen, the liver, and the small intestine with its little sidekick the appendix—alongside a string of lymph nodes. As a lean fifteen-year-old, I was not yet housing the five pounds of fat that move into the neighborhood as we grow older and wider. An incision running the length of my abdomen just east of my navel would create a bare-naked view of these vital tissues to help track the farthest wanderings of the cancer. Visual observations of the abdominal nodes and organs, combined with a snip here and a snip there to be examined under a microscope by the pathologist, would provide the last pieces of the puzzle to stage the disease. The lower the stage number, the shorter and less intense the treatment, and the better the prognosis for survival.

The night before my admission to St. Jude for the laparotomy, I closed the door to my bedroom to secure privacy and posed in my bikini underwear in front of the mirror. I lovingly stroked my belly with the palm of my hand in a circular, clockwise motion. Round and round my hand went, forming an imaginary circle around my navel. As my fingers caressed the smooth landscape of my abdomen, I gazed into the mirror, cocking my head slightly sideways, working hard to conjure up the image of a belly with a slash down the middle.

In a softly audible voice, I whispered, "Good-bye." I was speaking to myself *and* to my invisible medical fairy godmother who was peering over my shoulder into the mirror with me. We bid farewell to my unmarred unit. The possible outcomes of the surgery— pain, discomfort, new signs of unwanted tumors— never crossed my mind.

This sacred communion was the first of many rituals over the coming years to detach myself from a body part slated for sacrifice to the insatiable cancer demons. Those hungry little bastards lusted after my personal belongings, but that evening before my first major surgery, I felt calmed by the ritual. I was as ready as I was ever going to be.

On January 25, 1971, I was admitted to room 106 of the twenty-room inpatient ward. In the larger scheme of tests and treatments the St. Jude staff was obligated to inflict on the inmates, an exploratory laparotomy was not a particularly torturous event. I was a novice, however, in crossing the rocky terrain of surgery's aftermath. I quickly learned that many of the steps toward relocating your center of gravity are challenging. Yet it was enlightening to discover how the human body and psyche can endure a steady stream of unpleasantries.

As I lay in the hospital bed after the surgery, it soon became clear that I was no longer in Kansas. I tried to turn myself over from my back to my left side. Yowee! A three-hundred-pound linebacker was holding me down while his buddy belted me a good one in the tummy.

I soon became acutely aware of my abdominal muscles. These typically shy workhorses do their job in silence, allowing us to twist and bend. But they were blocking the surgeon's eagle-eyed view of the targeted tissues. In those days, no gentle parting could open up his line of vision. The surgeon had to slice through my abdominal muscles to get to the rolling landscape of my internal organs. But severed muscles cause intense pain.

I pushed the little brown button at the end of the cable lying over the bedrail. The nurse, affectionately known to me as Wonder Woman, materialized in a flash at my bedside.

"I need to turn over, but it hurts to move," I muttered as pitifully as I could.

"We can take care of that," Wonder Woman said, which I soon learned was doublespeak for Demerol is on the way! "Would you like for me to help you turn over first?"

"Mmmm, yes, please."

She gently slid both her hands under the left side of my lower back and very tenderly rolled the dead weight from my back to my side. She left me alone to feel the momentary relief from my dislodged body parts.

A minute later she was back. "I've got a shot that will take care of the pain. It'll just be a stick." Hovering over the bed, she pulled the sheet off and pulled my hospital gown up to expose my thigh. "Here comes the stick."

Wonder Woman joined the ranks of my trusted allies. The shot was not bad. The next few minutes were bliss. The shot contained fairy dust that permeated every corner of my body, relaxing even the tiniest of muscles. I became nothing more than a bodiless head nestled deliriously in my pillow. An epiphany filled the light, airy space where my thick fifteen-year-old brain had been.

Suddenly I had an insight. Despite what most people think, our hard-sought image of who we perceive ourselves to be has little to do with our physical bodies. We allow the body to masquerade as ourselves when, in reality, the meat of our being is all in our heads! Pretty intense stuff for a freshly budding teen.

As I loosened the reins on my self-image, a great swell of empathy for drug addicts percolated in my bobbed head. I now understood how someone could lose himself to illegally obtained substances. My head-on-a-pillow felt no fear of this newfound kinship with addicts. Peace, love, and understanding poured forth for everyone who relied on drugs for relief from their pain. Then I drifted off.

Room 106 was like every other room on the St. Jude inpatient unit. Adorning the hospital rooms was not a high priority for the much-needed research dollars. A bed, a chair, a nightstand, a hospital tray, a clock, and me—these were the contents of the room. It looked like an advertisement from the Hospital Depot discount catalog. Metal and Formica in the cheery colors of brown and gray were the materials of choice. No technological advances, such as a telephone or television, were allowed to consume Danny and Rose Marie's hard-earned dollars.

The only luxuries of this home away from home were two windows, and the views out of these windows were the semicolon in my daily sentence of life in room 106. Glimpses of the world beyond my room formed an essential link that I needed. One window faced the lawn. The opposite window faced the inpatient hallway. This three-by-four-foot piece of clear glass framed a flurry of indoor activity. Gray metal blinds controlled the view, and the blinds were often raised throughout the day to provide a distraction.

The hall window started about halfway up the wall, and when I lay in bed facing it, all I could see was a parade of doctors and nurses from the hips up. They always seemed to be in a hurry, rushing to their next urgent task, like actors in a St. Jude rendition of *General Hospital*.

A gurney floating by was not an uncommon sight, and because I couldn't see the gurney's legs, it looked as though the patients were suspended on a magic carpet. Viewing hours for St. Jude *General Hospital* were limited, though. A couple of times each day, the blinds were shut tightly for one of two purposes, either to help create the kind of darkness that nurtures a deep slumber, or to shield us innocent young'uns from our recently departed neighbors.

One night, they forgot to close the blinds. As I lay on my favorite left side staring out the window, drowsy from the Demerol-induced ups and downs of the day, a gurney strolled past the window. The passenger was unusually still. The feet came into view first. The body and head, and then the chauffeur, were not far behind. Yet the cast and plot were different tonight. The floating body was covered with a sheet from toe to head. The masked head was just passing outside my viewing screen when I realized what I was seeing.

No one was in my room with me at the time. I didn't move a muscle as I continued to stare at the vacant hall. I mulled over the outcome of this episode. No dramatic guiding light shone down on me, not at that moment anyway. My eyes were fastened to the window. The latest shot of Demerol began to wear off, and my unforgiving bruises snapped my dulled psyche to attention. I looked at the clock and sank into a funk. I had almost an hour to go before the usual four hours between shots had elapsed. Discomfort was creeping outward from some untouchable space inside my abdomen. I could not take my eyes off the clock, willing my glare to force the hand to the next hour.

Oh, heck, I thought. *I'm calling Wonder Woman now. Maybe she'll cave in to my pitiful pleas.* I pushed the button that magically brought her forth.

"I'm hurting again. The medicine has worn off."

"I'll be back with a shot in a few minutes," she said, unconcerned that I was forty-five minutes shy of the next green light. As I closed my eyes to patiently await my savior, the god of Demerol, I began to say the Sh'ma, the Jewish prayer of prayers.

"Sh'ma Yisrael Adonai Eloheinu Adonai Echad. Baruch sheim k'vod malchutoh l'olam vaed. V'ahavta eit Adonai Elohehcha b'chol . . ."

Tears rolled down my face as I reached out for a tangible connection to something infinitely larger than myself. "God, please get me though this. *Please.* Get me out of here! And while you're at it, would you please get me a decent boyfriend?"

Sadly, this is no joke. I actually included the latter request in my bargaining with God. Danny Thomas asked for hope and direction. I asked for a boyfriend.

To help guarantee delivery of a high-quality product, I added, "Give me a life after Hodgkin's with a good-looking, cool boyfriend, and I will say the Sh'ma every day for the rest of my life."

Desperation can take us down a crooked path. I was five-five, ninety pounds, as pale and droopy as the dreary curtains hanging in room 106. I looked like an anorexia nervosa patient who has not yet found her way into therapy. I had a snowball's chance in hell to attract the interest of a suitable candidate. But at that moment, the request seemed appropriate in my dialogue with the Almighty. "Just give me the goods, and I'll deliver," I promised.

Wonder Woman came back quickly to save the day. I knew the routine well by now. Off came the sheet. Up went my hospital gown. Ouch. Relief.

A young woman cannot live on Demerol alone, though. Food not only nourishes vital organs, but also helps quell the need for stimulation of the senses. Regular fixes of colorful, tasty flesh and flora keep the longings of our tongues and bellies satiated. Delirium sets in when these longings are not satisfied. After a few days with no food, save the hummingbird feed flowing into my IV and a few offerings of juice and cola, I saw visions of thick, juicy roast beef, mashed potatoes, and green beans lurking everywhere.

My stomach was starting to rumble. Rumbling was good. The audible ranting and raving of my stomach was the high sign the doctors were awaiting to free my GI tract from isolation. During the initial stupor from the anesthesia and pain medication, the muscles lining the walls of my stomach and intestines had assumed a relaxed posture along with the rest of my body, so they were unable to perform the rocking and rolling necessary to move food on down the line. But now my stomach was finally awakening from its slumber.

Having been alerted to the impending arrival of my first dinner, I was sitting up in bed, anxiously awaiting the feast. The nurse's aide slipped into the room balancing my tray in the air over her shoulder. "Here we are!" She demonstrated her mastery of the quarter-pivot-and-slide maneuver that gently lands the food onto the bedside hospital table. She adjusted the height of the table, pushing it over the bed, and stood there for a moment. Then she kindly removed the tops covering the array of containers.

"I know you're hungry. Give us a buzz if you need anything else." With that, she dashed out to complete her other deliveries.

I surveyed the tray. A neat arrangement of cylindrical vessels in the three primary food colors of the day had been placed before me: a cup of brown beef bouillon, a tumbler of golden apple juice, and a bowl of red Jell-O. Much to my surprise, the traces of beef flavor in the bouillon exploded on my bereft taste buds. I might as well have been eating steak tartare. And ooohhh—the joy of Jell-O! This divine, slippery cherry goodness was rich with the flavor and texture I was craving. Hats off to the chef. The meal could not have been more scrumptious. I was spoon-fed a lesson in the value of the simple, and sometimes well-disguised, pleasures of life.

This sensual experience was made all the more satisfying by the lonely routine of life on the St. Jude inpatient ward. No friends came to visit me, or more accurately, no friends my age managed to get back to the inpatient wing. Jeff and Jerry showed up one day unannounced, only to be met in the hospital lobby by Mickey, my brother-in-law, who turned them away.

"She's not allowed to have any visitors," he informed them kindly, but sternly.

They didn't come back. Friends couldn't call either since there was no phone in the room. They called my parents at home, however, and always heard the same response from my mother: "She's getting better. Nothing to worry about. She can't have visitors right now. She needs rest and shouldn't be exposed to germs that could cause an infection."

They were on the outside, and I was on the inside. As I learned later, whoever got the latest news on my progress activated the Minda Underground News Network, and by the end of the day, every teen who cared would have the scoop.

Along with my family, the St. Jude staff went out of their way to fill the void. When you joined the privileged ranks of St. Jude patients, you were protected in a womb of holistic care that included not only the medical staff assigned to you, but also administrative and research staff involved in your case. Rarely a day went by without a visit from Dr. Granoff, the researcher, teacher, mentor, and father of a friend who chaired the Virology/Molecular Biology Department.

Danny and Marlo Thomas, regular visitors to the hospital, strolled the halls popping into patients' rooms when appropriate. My mother suspected that the burden of all these children's cliff-hanger lives took a toll on Danny. She recalls he rarely smiled. His comedic calling had not enabled him to find levity in the tenuous young lives. No doubt, though, his larger-than-life presence lifted the spirits of patients, family, and staff.

On Thursday, January 28, 1971, my uterus began its virgin menstrual cleansing. I was fifteen, so I was a late bloomer. Before that, the cancer had consumed too many calories to allow the deposition of enough fat for maturation of my reproductive parts. By now, though, twenty-five days of radiation had put a damper on the voracious appetites of the cancerous cells. The unwanted critters were under siege, cut off from their food supplies and freeing up the calories to pad my gangly frame with a bit of fat.

My medical record documented the momentous occasion. The notes from the 3:00 to 11:00 shift read:

[Minda] *has begun her menstrual period with small amount of bleeding.*

Aren't I fortunate? How many women have professional documentation of the day and time their menstrual cycle officially started? I was ecstatic to be finally one of *the women*. My official initiation into the tribe was long overdue.

By day seven after Surgery Number One, the job of healing was well under way. Dr. M., a resident, came into my room to remove the staples that closed my incision. The term *staples* was a euphemism. Staple removers better described these small metal clamps holding my abdomen together.

Dr. M. sat next to me on the bed as he leaned over my belly to begin the task. He pulled back the sheet, and I raised my hospital gown to expose the work surface. He looked up and smiled at me. "This shouldn't take too long." I think his terse words of encouragement were meant to reassure himself more than me.

With a pair of needle-nosed pliers, which probably had some innocuous-sounding medical name like "surgical disbanders," he bent the middle of the head of each clamp so the teeth backed out of my skin. Stinging throbs shot through my flesh as, one by one, he removed the clamps, leaving fourteen small open wounds on each side of the gash on my once smooth belly. With each subsequent loosening of the jaws of the clamps, my tears welled. Dr. M. stayed focused on my belly, seemingly unaware of the pain he was inflicting.

When he finished, he looked up at me, pleased as punch that he had completed the task with no mishaps. "Anything else I can do for you?"

I paused for a moment, glaring at him intently through my tears, and screamed, "Get out of my room, and don't ever come back!"

He was stunned. "I'm sorry. We're done, and you won't have to do this again." (It turned out he was wrong.) Then he dashed out.

A couple of hours later, Dr. J. came by to bid us his formal adieu and lay out the next steps. He sat on my bed and scolded me in the lighthearted manner the St. Jude docs and nurses practiced so well. "You really scared Dr. M. He's decided he no longer wants to be a doctor!"

By that time, the pain had already diminished, and I felt joyous about my impending release. But I wasn't sorry I screamed at Dr. M.

Dr. J. presented the St. Jude team's perspective of my diagnosis and the plan for the next phase of treatment. Fortunately, all the pathology reports from the surgical biopsies came back negative. There were no signs of cancer anywhere except in my neck and chest. I was labeled Stage IIA (out of IV). *Stage II* indicated two node-involved regions on the same side of the diaphragm. It meant the absence of at least one of three clinical symptoms: drenching night sweats, more than ten percent weight loss, and unexplained fever.

Now that the surgery was over and the staging was set, just one more simple procedure stood between me and outpatient status—my first chemo treatment.

chapter three

1971, FEBRUARY

Mother Nature can be a devious queen, hiding her most valuable treasures from the masses. From raw diamonds to the unsightly, yet delectable morel mushroom, she dresses her precious resources in deceptive designs. She is particularly conniving when it comes to her healing balms for the wounded, sequestering curative secrets deep within the complex chemical structure of plants. For centuries, these medicinal gold mines have remained untouched. One by one, though, the buried treasures have been unearthed by explorers who miraculously stumble upon these natural gifts.

Yet Mother Nature has stiff competition these days. The pharmaceutical gods have infiltrated her database, creating ingenious treatments for some of the deadliest diseases. I became a disciple, devoted to these latter-day saviors, when I began my first round of chemotherapy.

Eli Lilly, a dominant pharmaceutical god, sniffed out one of the Mother's most potent secrets in the 1950s when exploring a cure for cancer. Master Lilly tapped into the sap of the common periwinkle, a plant with a

widely dispersed family of cousins living in far corners
of the earth. Used for centuries as a folk remedy for a
variety of ailments including diabetes and anxiety, this
low-lying ground cover with vibrant purple flowers
contains alkaloids that stop the reproduction of fast-
growing lymphoma cells dead in their tracks. The
original source of this powerful chemical was the rosy
periwinkle of Madagascar, later produced synthetically
and called vincristine, after the botanical genus *Vinca*.

Vincristine became both my best friend and my
worst enemy. On February 3, 1971, I received my first
intravenous doses of what I refer to as "CanceRid," a
vial of vincristine followed by a vial of cyclophosphamide, another potent cancercide. My body
seemed unimpressed by this first treatment. I tolerated
it well and went home on a pass, with orders to return
the next morning at 10:00 for my official transfer from
inpatient to outpatient status. The next day, my GI tract
staged its first revolt.

Some folks tolerate chemotherapy with minimal
side effects. My GI tract took to the chemo like a
vegetarian to an all-beef hot dog. On the drive back to
the hospital, my breakfast reappeared, the first of
hundreds of attempts by my GI tract to let me and the
doctors know she was not a happy camper.

The chemical tools of torture were non-
discriminating tyrants, making a beeline for all my
rapidly dividing cells—the cancerous cells as well as the
cells of my GI tract, hair, and blood. These normal cells
paid the price for being antsy to procreate, resulting in
the loss of my hair and plummeting red and white
blood cells counts. The dying cells in the lining of my
stomach and intestines revolted with violent nausea.
My stomach staged a wretched, rhythmic rebellion,

forcing me to heave until there was nothing more than a frenetic muscular reaction yielding only air and tears.

The diagnosis of Stage II Hodgkin's mandated a one-year siege of chemical warfare. The CanceRid was to be dripped into my veins over a period of twelve months, starting with an outpatient schedule of one time per week. Every Thursday, my mother accompanied me to St. Jude for the exhausting ritual. As with most cancer treatment clinics, St. Jude's Torture Chamber was euphemistically known as "the medicine room."

In those years, the medicine room reflected a constrained budget. When it was time for my treatment, they called my name, and Mom and I were escorted from the front lobby to a sparsely adorned room filled with a couple of gurneys, a few padded chairs and wooden rockers, and several sick kids who rarely spoke to each other. Parents, mostly mothers, were present to hold their children's hands. No TV, not even a small one, was available for diversion. It wouldn't have mattered for us kids anyway, because the daytime offerings by the only three networks were the melodramas of *As the World Turns*, *General Hospital*, and *The Guiding Light*.

Also missing from the early days of group chemotherapy were curtains to spare each of us from our comrades' misery. One after the other, we spewed our guts out. Unlike self-conscious adults, we quickly adapted and were immune to embarrassment, maybe because we were all in the same rickety boat.

Memories of the post-infusion vomiting, vomiting, and more vomiting still underscore my entire St. Jude experience. The most startling contrast between then and now was the missing antiemetic weapon to suppress the nausea. Phenergan suppositories were available, but were offered only at the worst of times because they had unwanted side effects. On most days, a stick of Wrigley's spearmint gum was the only peace offering to my enraged GI tract.

To this day, when offered gum, I always ask, "What kind is it?" If it's spearmint or anything close, I reply with a blunt "no thanks." The harsh tone of my response to an innocuous offer sometimes necessitates a more elaborate explanation, and the unsuspecting soul is usually quite polite as I unload *The Tale of the Chewing Gum Aversion*.

A passing whiff of a certain type of hair conditioner can also drag me back to the St. Jude medicine room. Today we accept baldness as a necessary evil of cancer chemotherapy. Cancer equals baldness. Baldness equals cancer. We are so well indoctrinated that when we see a bald woman, we assume she has cancer, and our hearts go out to her. But the balding doesn't occur overnight. It can take a few weeks before the CanceRid goes into effect.

I was blessed with strong, glossy hair. "Shining, gleaming, streaming . . . My Hair!" Along with my pert breasts and my daily recitation of the Sh'ma, my hair was essential to my Decent Boyfriend pact with God. One day, after the second or third treatment, I was prepping my hair for a much-needed outing with friends when suddenly a web of my luscious waves caught in the bristles of my hair brush and came loose.

I gasped. Then I stroked my hair again to make sure I was not adding two and two to make nine. Yep, the time had come. Dozens of precious hairs did not even whimper as they fell. Would they all go down that easily?

Cream rinse came to the rescue. I could not get enough of Suave cream rinse. I used large quantities to minimize the tangles when I combed. Just a few strokes were needed after a shampoo to detangle my mop. These regular fixes of cetyl and stearyl alcohols in the cream rinse left me with a Pavlovian response that still wields its powerful effect. Whenever I open a bottle of cream rinse, the screeching violins from Alfred Hitchcock's *Psycho* sound in my head, and nausea blooms in my gut. My salivary glands squirt streams of saliva under my tongue. As the nausea becomes more intense, the *eeek, eeek, eeek!* gets louder and louder until I manage to put the top back on the bottle, sealing off the offensive fumes. And then the nausea is gone.

Cream rinse was not my only weapon to ward off the loss of my beautiful locks. I discovered Pssst, a dry-cleaning hair product whose popularity was short-lived. Pssst was basically baby powder in a spray can. A few sprays soaked up the oil and seemed to delay the destruction from a full shampoo. Three sprays—pssst, pssst, pssst—and a tightly woven braid, and I was good to go for several days. It didn't take me long to realize that a few shakes of Johnson and Johnson's baby powder did the same thing.

By minimally washing and combing my hair, I believed I was postponing the inevitable. The inevitable never came. Even though my thick hair dwindled to an anemic braid of three thin ropes, the hair loss came to an abrupt halt in the middle of the CanceRid treatments. It was as though someone flipped the off switch, and the hair follicles regained their sturdy grip. Still, I continued to treat the hair survivors with gentle care, living in fear that the switch would be tripped on again.

One new friend, the Wig, waited patiently atop a faceless mannequin head sitting on my dresser. My mother and I had searched long and hard for the lifelike fall, traipsing in and out of every wig shop in Memphis. When it was apparent the CanceRid's effect on my head was over, the Wig and her pedestal were stuffed in the closet—just in case. Fortunately, that case never came.

A footnote for those of you inspired to try Pssst. In the 1970s, a society obsessed with cleanliness could not adjust to a product designed to promote dirty hair. This created insurmountable marketing challenges for Pssst. Recently, it has been repackaged and promoted as a hair product for *camping, after sports, and when ill.*

Side effect number three of the life-saving chemo was weight loss. As a cancer-ridden teenager whose intrusive guest had first dibs on my fuel sources, I didn't exactly have mounds of stored fat to see me through. I began the CanceRid with a pitiful ninety pounds of muscle, bones, and bodily fluids, and much to the dismay of the doctors, my weight hovered at that meager level for several months. Still, my appetite severely suffered from the ongoing rebellions of my GI tract.

Jewish mothers know the perfect antidote for wasting, and mine heard the call. Ice cream, shrimp cocktails, chocolate Nutrament. She also bought some funky, thin-sliced roast beef rolled up in a jar like a specimen in formaldehyde. You name the craving, my mother was there to provide, regardless of the conflict with Jewish dietary laws.

Some evenings she patiently fed me spoonful by spoonful. "Here's a bite for Sharon. Here's a bite for Carol. Let's take a bite for Reva. And let's not forget Paul [my favorite Beatle]."

We would giggle as we conjured up to whom the next bite would be dedicated. Like a picky two-year-old, I consumed the entire plate before I knew it! Clearly, I was screaming out for my mother's help. Her gentle feeding offered with love was just the nourishment the doctor ordered for my weakened body and soul.

A month after the first four CanceRid treatments, the side effects worsened, and a few of my nerves joined the revolt. First my fingertips began to tingle, then they went numb. I woke up in the middle of the night with leg cramps. Next my entire body reacted with an extreme lethargy. It took all the energy I could muster to hobble into the waiting room each Thursday and collapse into a chair. Contorting my lean limbs into a folded yogic chair twist, I drifted into a drug-induced stupor. In this quasi-hibernation, I awaited the call of my name for the next treatment. My mother was always by my side.

Fortunately, St. Jude altered my treatment. *Stay the course* was not the mantra of the era, because the well-tested recipes matching the most effective treatment to your specific type and stage of cancer had not yet been refined. St. Jude was desperately searching for the best combination of drugs to stop the invader while keeping the host alive, and they knew vincristine was the culprit of my wear and tear. So for four treatments they loaded their guns with cyclophosphamide only. They still felt I needed vincristine, however, so about a month later, they reinstated it at one-fourth the original dosage.

During all this upheaval festering in my body during the first few months of treatment, one life-altering, positive event occurred, unnoticed at the time. I uncovered this information years later while reviewing medical records for this book.

Dr. Omar Hustu, a gentle, soft-spoken physician, entered my life the day after my first chemo treatment. Varied images of dozens of doctors have filled the files in my memory bank since contact with Dr. Hustu decades ago. Yet his sparkling brown eyes, bushy Groucho-like eyebrows, and serene demeanor still elicit a uniquely healing warmth – a rare memory from my travels through the health care maze. As a radiation oncologist, Dr. Hustu was charged with determining where and how much more radiation I should receive. He recorded his decision in my St. Jude medical chart on February 4, 1971. Twenty-nine years later I discovered this entry:

> *In spite of findings I'm incline* [sic] *to treat para-aortic area because of large and low mediast. mass. On the other hand—by the same facts—do not feel justified (with its implications) in treating the pelvis in this patient.*   O. Hustu

Time stood still as I was taken back to the day and the decision that allowed my daughter to be born. As I read the entry, I was both horrified and ecstatic to realize my sweet Dr. Hustu, in one bold decision, stopped the walrus from snuffing out the most valued treasure of my life.

Shea, oh, dear daughter Shea, please cherish this life you almost missed . . .

Dr. Hustu has passed, but his thoughtful balance of the use of killing tools with quality of life lives on with the current generation of St. Jude practitioners—and my daughter.

Back in the realm of the latest, greatest 1971 path to wellness, the CanceRid treatments were combined with an additional twenty-five days of radiation. The cycle of St. Jude to school and back again became routine.

Monday:	Radiation at 8a.m. followed by school.
Tuesday:	Radiation at 8a.m. followed by school.
Wednesday:	Radiation at 8a.m. followed by school.
Thursday:	No school, chemo treatment, vomiting, bed.
Friday:	Home sick.
Weekend:	Rest and recovery.

To help assure I did not fall behind in my schoolwork, Miss Griffith, the guidance counselor, assigned a sharp-witted whiz kid to tutor me in Algebra II. Barry Sulkin, the tutor, was two years my senior. Although he was *far* inferior in math to his tutoree, this distant cousin would later play a vital role in my health, healing, and overall well-being. More on this later.

Radiation treatments ended in March. Then in mid-May, while I was walking up the stairs to the second floor for Spanish class, a piercing pain sliced through my abdomen. I went on up the stairs, casually continuing my conversation with Laurie and suffering in silence to avoid drawing attention.

At that point, I was living a double life. At school, I was Minda, the teen cancer poster child who was valiantly maintaining a heroic degree of normalcy amidst an abnormal lifestyle. At home and St. Jude, Minda was the sickly daughter, sister, niece, patient who was physically fragile and dependent on others for emotional and medical support.

The abdominal cramping waxed and waned over the next few days, but like labor pains, the bouts of sharp throbbing steadily increased in severity. Was I giving birth to a new tumor? By day four, the alien had taken command of my abdomen and was no longer holding back. In laywoman's terms, it hurt like hell. My appetite and bowel movements withered away with the escalating waves of cramping.

St. Jude staff came to the rescue. With their white Superman capes, they promptly diagnosed the problem, halted my chemo treatment, and admitted me to inpatient room 107. Obstruction from intestinal adhesions was not unusual after abdominal surgery, and after my earlier laparotomy, my gut had generated scar tissue to heal the wounds, sometimes in unwanted places. My scar tissue was described as a *piano string adhesive band* blocking the midsection of my small intestine.

A tube shoved down one of my nostrils into my gut was the first line of defense. Using a tool reminiscent of the Roto-Rooter, the doctors hoped to avoid surgery by sucking out the stomach and bile secretions, reducing gas buildup, and in the process, decompressing my stressed bowel. My GI tract waged war with the Piano String (and perhaps the tube), causing me to vomit again and again.

The tube hanging out of my nose seemed to be doing its job, with almost three cups of dark green muck suctioned off in the first day. But Piano String was holding on for dear life as the vomiting, cramping, and suctioning continued for another day. In the wee hours of the following night, the tides started to turn.

"Yes, I passed some gas!" I declared to the nurse. This was a sign the bottleneck might be breaking loose. Let the traffic flow!

A few hours later, my spirits were dampened as the green sewage came forth again—from both ends. It was as disgusting as Linda Blair's coming-out party in *The Exorcist*. I ejected the horrid-looking pea soup from my mouth at the same time Mr. Rooter siphoned off a respectable quantity into the bottle beside my bed. My mood sank to an all-time low.

Seems depressed—is uncommunicative and smiles very rarely, wrote the nurse in the medical chart.

I don't get it. I had a bruised nostril from a piece of plastic shoved through the oh-so-small opening of my oh-so-not-petite nose; my throat was sore from simultaneously accommodating the plastic tubing *and* the vomiting; my intestinal muscles were working overtime to rid me of the rank contents; and there was the coolest outfit ever hanging at home in the closet for the dance the following Saturday night. Were they expecting Beaver Cleaver's cheerful grin? I was *not* having a good time.

A few weeks earlier, life had been looking up. God had stepped up to the plate to keep her part of the Sh'ma/Cool Boyfriend contract. One night when I was feeling well enough to be back on the social scene, the boyfriend had magically appeared with a greasy mushroom pizza at Pete and Sam's Restaurant. Steve had noticed me from across the room, apparently had liked what he saw, and had come over to my table to introduce himself. It did not take us long to find common ground. As fate would have it, Steve was the son of Dr. Salky, who had diagnosed my Hodgkin's. Steve was a cool dude, and I was happy.

But now, in this duel with Piano String, was God now reneging on her bargain? Would I have to offer up another body part to get out of here in time to wear the mod outfit on my upcoming date with Steve?

On day three, they removed the tube, and I was *talking and smiling* and *in much better spirits*, according to my chart. The most important question on my mind was, *When is this nightmare going to end so I can go to the party?* Unfortunately, more vomiting ensued, and by nightfall, the tube was reinserted.

Day four. Piano String was winning the battle. It was time to attack the scoundrel the old-fashioned way—with a scalpel. Slice Number Two was made right on top of Slice Number One. Fourteen new staples were inserted into my tender belly, and by 12:30 that afternoon, I was back in room 107 sans Piano String. The tube and green muck were back on the agenda for the next couple of days, and as usual, Mom, Dad, Reva, and Mickey stayed by my side. Over the next week, I lay recovering in my room, assisted by the luxurious accoutrements of hospital food, gastric tubes and sleep deprivation.

Then one day, *That Girl* appeared at my bedside, larger than life (though quite svelte). A photographer captured my visit with Marlo Thomas. She was Danny and Rose Marie's eldest, and an Emmy award-winning actress in her fifth season with her popular TV series. In the eight-by-ten photo, delivered to my home later that month, Marlo stood by my bed spellbindingly attractive and poised. The patient, on the other hand, looked... well, like a cancer kid, emaciated and pitifully adorned with a tube running out of her schnozzle. The woeful image of Patient 2410, minus Marlo, appeared on the front of the next St. Jude fundraising appeal with the caption *CONTRIBUTIONS PAY TO KEEP THESE CHILDREN ALIVE!*

St. Jude dollars worked their magic. I healed from Surgery Number Two on schedule and was discharged on June 3, 1971—six days *after* the formal dance. My party skirt and blouse were cotton, black and tan with splashes of red in geometric patterns, with hints of Egyptian and East Indian influences. The sleeveless blouse was angled at the shoulders and gathered at the collar. The outfit hung in my closet for years—unworn. Never again did I fit into a size three. I still haven't gotten over *not* being able to wear that smartly designed outfit, whose details I remember like an impassioned one-night stand.

Yet that outfit inspired an act of kindness. Before the dance, I'd been lamenting the destiny of my skirt and blouse to Barry, my math tutor. Touched by my situation, he rejected the social norms of renting a tuxedo when he attended the formal dance. Instead, he wore his own suit and donated the sixty dollars to St. Jude.

Upon release from the hospital, I graduated to a reduced schedule for CanceRid treatments, one visit every other week. As intimate as I had become with my St. Jude family, I relished the thought of creating more space between me and my codependents. I was ready to jump to Step Twelve, though we were probably on about Step Six with ten more months of therapy to go. Two treatments later and almost seven months after my diagnosis, the medical record states:

ASYMPTOMATIC. NO EVIDENCE OF ACTIVE DISEASE AT THIS TIME
                        ~ July 8, 1971

There was more good news. With my mother's cajoling to "eat more," my weight crept up to a hefty 108 pounds. By the end of 1971, I had climbed from no-man's-land all the way up the growth chart to a reasonably healthy thirtieth percentile. Out of ten "average" teens my age and height, two would weigh less than me.

With all this great news of robust poundage, I was rewarded with a full dosage of both vincristine and cyclophosphamide—because even though there were no signs of active cancer, the protocol required additional chemotherapy to assure destruction of any hidden cells. But I could have told them my still delicate body was not ready for this much company.

Two weeks later, I arrived at the clinic with my calf muscles taking a rigid stand of protest, cramping unpredictably. My pilot light was barely glimmering, dulled by overwhelming lethargy. The doctors took mercy on me, and during the next few treatments, they gradually decreased the vincristine until it was eliminated altogether. As the year 1971 drew to a close, I headed into the home stretch with only three more treatments to go.

1972

I guess my GI tract was sensing this part of our journey was almost over. Like a naughty, neglected child, it longed for more of the care and attention it got when wreaking havoc. So in January, 1972, more scar tissue cropped up in my gut. Hoping to avoid another major surgery, the doctors placed me on an oral medication and sent me home.

It got better before it got worse. Then ten days after the initial sign of trouble, the pain became constant and unbearable. More and more of the partially digested portions of my meals were coming out the entrance because the exit door was closing fast. When I could take it no longer, my parents rushed me to St. Jude, and around 1:00 a.m., I was deposited in room 116 of the inpatient ward.

In a last-ditch effort to avoid abdominal Surgery Number Three, the docs called in my good friend again, the nasogastric tube. When the nurse walked in with the tube in her hand, I almost mustered up the wherewithal to heal myself. Unfortunately, I had not yet mastered the powers of self-healing. *Here we go again*, I thought.

The first tube went down relatively easily followed by a dash of Demerol in the IV to relieve the discomforts. I seemed to be on my way.

Not so easy. A kink in the plumbing. The tube was pulled out and replaced with another one. My GI tract gave in a little—just enough to give the doctors cause for hope—and then it revolted again. The volume coming out of my mouth exceeded what the Roto-Rooter was suctioning into the bottle next to the bed.

Day three. Time for heavier artillery. The nurse pulled the tube out of my nose just long enough for me to take a few unobstructed breaths. The next game plan involved Roto-Rooter Plus—a tube with a small rubber balloon at the end filled with a dollop of a heavy metal.

"You've got to be kidding me. You're not going to put that in my nose?"

I whimpered in horror as I contemplated the bag fitting through my swollen nasal passage. The inside of my nostril had grown smaller over the past couple of days as it had snuggled around the last two tubes.

"Sorry, dear. Let's just get it over with. It won't take long."

The nurse's job was probably harder than mine. Imagine shoving a bag through an orifice half its size. I laid my head back on the pillow as her hand approached my nose. Push. Push. The petroleum-covered bag slipped surprisingly fast through my nostril and landed at the back of my throat. I gagged, shut my eyes tightly, took a big gulp, and swallowed the rubber bag before I had a chance to think about it.

It was to no avail. My arrogant GI tract held on, and the next day the doctors sent me off to surgery for Round Three. If we had only known, prior to the first laparotomy, I could have passed on to the surgeons my sewing expertise of installing zippers and bound button holes. But it was not meant to be. The surgeons did the best they could, but after my third teenage field trip to the OR, I looked like the victim of a knife fight. I had a jagged quarter-inch-wide scar running the length of my belly, bordered on both sides by a row of white psychedelic puncture wounds from the staples.

As with Surgery Number Two, the operation went smoothly, and the obstruction in my intestine was clipped away with no complications. Toward the end of this final episode of *The Trilogy of the Laps*, I received permission to go up the hall to use the pay phone. I had a strong hankering to talk to Steve, my boyfriend—you know, the cool dude who was part of the contract. (I had not gone through all of this hullabaloo for nothing). I was feeling pretty spunky, so I scuttled on my own two spindly legs while I pushed the wheelchair in front of me. At that point, the wheelchair was a prop, not for me, but for the IV still attached to my hand. So me and my IV went on an adventure.

The phone booth was in another hallway adjoining the inpatient unit. It was evening, and like a museum after visiting hours, the halls were pitch-black and deserted. With the exception of the inpatient ward, St. Jude was a daytime operation. For a few brief minutes, I was busting out of prison to explore the hinterlands and connect with a friend on the outside. My heart was pounding, to the beat of love, not fear, as I slid into the seat in the phone booth. Of course, the wheelchair would not fit, so I left the phone booth door cracked open, just enough for my IV tubing.

I assumed we were alone, but before I had a chance to complete the dialing of Steve's number, I suddenly felt a strong pull on my IV. Someone was trying to run off with my wheelchair! I shoved open the phone booth door, poked my head out, and discovered a scene straight from a Laurel and Hardy script. A maintenance person was pushing the "abandoned" wheelchair out of the middle of the hallway, unaware a patient was attached. I leaped out of the booth in time to keep the needle from pulling loose.

"Excuse me, ma'am," I blurted out. "Me and it are still attached." I pointed to the wheelchair and the IV.

She looked as though she had just seen a ghost. "Why, I'm so sorry. I was going to put this wheelchair where it belonged. I didn't hurt you now, did I?" *Everyone* at St. Jude was nice, *always* treating patients like royalty.

"No, ma'am. I'm fine. Just here to call a friend." I made sure she didn't think I was out gallivanting around, trying to cause trouble.

She shook her head and left. I think I scared her. I was shaken, too. I decided to punt the call and go back to my safe haven, room 116.The brief stint into the outside world had exhausted me. I staggered back to my room, crawled into bed, and fell right to sleep.

Three days later, on day fourteen of this latest bonding time with my St. Jude family, I was sent home for two weeks of rest and recuperation before returning to school.

More than three weeks of gastrointestinal upheaval put a damper on Mother Matilda's North Beach Diet. I weighed in around one hundred pounds, and for the next few weeks, I suffered through milk shakes, steaks, potato chips, Nestle Crunch bars, and endless episodes of *Mayberry, RFD*. Times were rough.

In March, I resumed the CanceRid treatments with cyclophosphamide only. On April 6, 1972, my treatment for Hodgkin's disease, Stage IIA, came to an end. Four hundred and twenty nine days after the chemo began, the nurse inserted the IV needle into my arm for the final treatment. I ejected the next few meals for what I hoped would be the last time. I was worn out, but riding high on the excitement of Life after Cancer. I had finally won the jack pot—winner takes all. Life. During those seventeen months, the calendar said I'd turned one year older—from fifteen to sixteen. But my heart, mind, and soul had aged decades, with many hard-earned lessons that would shepherd me safely through the next few years.

Trauma comes in many shapes and sizes. But if the planets are aligned correctly, it leads to a precious wisdom. As you gaze through the fog and struggle to regain your focus, the nuggets of wisdom become evident bit by bit. You squint and squint as your view opens wider to a sparkling new awareness. I walked out those front glass doors of the old St. Jude after my last treatment with a patchwork quilt of rich and holy knowledge. I was joyful. I was connected. I was peaceful. I was alive. All in one moment. Every moment.

I had learned that truths are buried in paradoxes:
- Nothing is important. Everything is important.
- Don't sweat the small stuff. Find meaning in life's barest simplicities.
- Family and friends form the magic carpet that keeps us floating. It is up to you and you alone to stay grounded.
- Hold fast to and never lose sight of what matters. As Gumby, the green clay action figure, said, "It is important to be honest, it is important to be humble, but it is most important to be flexible."

I spent the final year of high school as any well-nourished teen—yakking on the phone, riding around in cars, partying at the homes of kids with absentee parents, while maintaining a studious profile and keeping my grade point average up. Before leaving for college, I had my fortune told at a party. A mysterious young hippy gazed at my hand, and then, without emotion, she said, "You won't live past twenty-seven years of age."

I didn't believe her. Certainly not. In August of 1973, I left Memphis for college, guided by my emerging wisdom but nagged by her prediction of doom.

chapter four

1974

Little Miss Fortune Teller, with her dire predictions of my death at twenty-seven, possessed the soothsaying skills of a broken clock. Nevertheless, her doomsday prophecy hung over my vulnerable psyche through a number of scares in the years leading up to that dreaded birthday.

The first scare occurred during my freshman year at Indiana University. In the winter of 1974, my fertile lymph system sprouted a swollen node in my neck. The persistent little bastard lingered long enough to frighten my body's three-headed guardian—my mother, my newest doctor at St. Jude, Dr. T, and myself. The wait-and-worry phase came and went. When the node remained swollen, it was time to act.

I called home to deliver the worrisome news and set plans in motion to return to Memphis for a visit with Dr. T. Just picking up the phone and making the long-distance connection with my parents brought me comfort. Mom said she would call St. Jude to make an appointment.

A few days after the travel plans had been made, I called her again. I was in tears, so upset that my sobbing and gasps were the only greeting my mother heard when she picked up the phone.

She disguised her own fretfulness to reassure me. "I'm so sorry, Minda. We're all really worried, but Dr. T. says it's probably nothing serious. She just needs to see you to make sure."

"But, Mom, you don't understand. I just found out I have a fifth row center seat for the Bob Dylan concert! We *have* to change the appointment!"

My mother was unable to reach across the generation gap to feel the gravity of my sorrow. From a mother's perspective, sacrificing a once-in-a-lifetime opportunity to see Bob Dylan from spittin' distance — at his first concert tour in eight years — did not climb to the top of her priority list.

I tried to explain: "Carol [my hall mate] won four seats. These are some of the most coveted tickets in the entire country!"

Carol had won the tickets in a mail order lottery, and in 1974, this was a novelty, an ingenious alternative to the box office mob scene for one of the most in-demand concerts in rock music history. Millions of people, over five percent of the US population, made requests for a seating in this twenty-one-city tour, and the fervor intensified as the announcement of the winners drew close. Carol hit the jackpot, scoring four of the best seats in the house. And one was for me.

Mom did not budge. I missed the concert, but won the more important lottery. As is often the case with the mysterious ways of the body, by the time I got to the St. Jude clinic, the swelling had disappeared. I traded Dylan up close and not so personal for peace of mind. It was worth it.

Toward the end of my freshman year, I had another minor scare. I contracted some of the most bull-headed genital warts this side of free love that the university doctors had ever seen. One wart was so big and oddly placed that my urine burned a hole right through the middle of it in a desperate attempt to find an exit. I mention this gruesome development because it was the grand finale to my breakaway year, the first year away from the medical and emotional support of home. Good job, Minda.

I returned home from college for the summer and was hospitalized for several days for a cleansing of my vagina. My mother doesn't remember the explanation she gave the neighbors for my hospitalization. But thirty-two years later, the *Commercial Appeal*, the esteemed Memphis daily, published this unseemly detail to the entire city because I had unwisely disclosed this information in an interview for an article highlighting the latent effects of childhood cancer treatment.

> "The cancer combined with the surgery, radiation and chemotherapy that saved her life set her up for the health problems that have stalked her since college. They include collapsed lungs, shingles, genital warts. . ."

> *Memphis Commercial Appeal,*
> October 29, 2006

My body and I navigated the rest of my undergraduate years rather smoothly. *Smoothly* excluded the trauma of being caught by my parents with a bag of pot and subsequently transferring to the "less radical" University of Tennessee.

During each of these death-defying years, I celebrated my birthday with a sigh of relief as I slipped by Little Miss Fortune Teller's rosy prediction. Actually, I had conjured up an idiotic theory that my risk of cancer was *lower* than my peers because the radiation and CanceRid had cleansed my body of *all* cancerous cells. Zap. Every mutant was gone. I was like a quart of ultra-pasteurized milk, whereas my friends were unpasteurized. This *Pasteurized Milk Theory* bolstered my confidence.

Anchoring my ride through the minor detours of those years was Barry, my high school math tutor. Remember him? After the cool guy Steve dumped me— on a positive note of *you have potential*— Barry got my heart to fluttering again. By my freshman year of college, our relationship had progressed from math tutor to close friend to long-distance lover. After his graduation from the University of Virginia, he joined me in Knoxville for my final two years of undergraduate education.

Barry and I pursued similarly crooked paths toward our Bachelor's degrees, abandoning our first majors for careers more suitable to our activist natures. For me, the nascent debate about the connection between our diets and cancer inspired a change of major from computer science to nutrition science. Barry's love of the outdoors (and rock and roll) led him away from the demanding chemical engineering major and toward a degree in environmental science with a minor in staging rock concerts.

After a tour of God's country from Colorado to Washington State searching for a new home in the wilder West, we made a 180-degree turn right back to the South, to the affordable, deciduously green hill country of Middle Tennessee.

1977

In 1977, at twenty-two and twenty-four years of age, we had the mature foresight to recognize the value of a home within driving distance from our parents, yet distant enough to prevent frequent visits. Nashville felt just right, with an eclectic music scene rooted amid thousands of acres of countryside not yet adulterated with urban sprawl.

We both landed jobs with the Tennessee Department of Public Health, Barry with the Water Quality Division and me with the Nutrition Division. Food and water. Between the two of us, we covered the basic sustenance of life. We settled into our heathen, common law relationship in a little log cabin in the woods outside Nashville. Life was mighty fine.

Then the garden in my lymph system began to grow. Plump little pods germinated—this time in my groin.

Since the Scare of 1974, I had developed a touchy relationship with the nodes in my neck and groin. I was scared to feel them, yet I couldn't keep my hands away from them. Every night, I sat in bed and contemplated whether to touch or not to touch. I eventually gathered the courage to act, gently rolling my fingertips over my groin. This trench harbored danger. The puny marbles came and went. Sometimes they were tender and sore, sometimes pain-free. I had been told that tender or sore were good signs, indicative of swelling in reaction to an infection, *not* cancer.

1978

In June, 1978, I went to the Vanderbilt Hospital Emergency Room with a raunchy case of the hives. The ER resident listened attentively as I told him my Hodgkin's history.

"Are you aware of these swollen nodes?" he asked after palpating my groin.

"Yes." I told him the saga of my on-again, off-again self-examinations.

"You should have these nodes biopsied right away. Do you want to have the biopsy done here or go back to St. Jude?"

He wasn't fooling around, posing a question without the option of no for an answer. Even though I knew he was a novice, his reaction threw my worry meter over the top, trumping my faith in the wait-and-see approach.

The resident left the room to obtain a second opinion, and a few minutes later he returned. "I talked with Vanderbilt's leading hematologist, Dr. John Flexner, and he concurred. The lymph nodes should be removed as soon as possible. When do you want to have this done?" He was proud of himself for making the right call.

"I better check with my doctors at St. Jude," I said, stalling for time. I promised I would have it checked out right away. The next week, Barry and I drove to Memphis to visit Dr. T.

She felt the nodes and was unimpressed. The nodes had not changed from the last visit, and the fact that they were rather soft led her to recommend continued observation. We returned home, and I tried to shove the fret into an inaccessible corner of my short-term recall.

Over the next few months, the lymph nodes waxed and waned, not unlike the moon, except my little moons did not have predictable lunar cycles. I resumed the nightly ritual of OLD—obsessive lymphnode disorder. I was never quite sure what I would find when I went exploring. Change or no change, though, the worry was always there. I learned to acknowledge the fear and then to turn it off for the night so I could rest at ease.

Meanwhile, in November, 1978, Barry and I took two grand steps toward legitimizing our alternative lifestyle. We bought a farm, and we got married. We secured the contract for the latter affair in short order before a local judge and his secretary. Barry accepted the fragility of my future better than I did, asserting he married me knowing I might not be around for the long haul. With our new home in the country, food (her job), water (his job), and our upstanding legal contract (marriage), we were hopeful the haul would be longer rather than shorter.

Soon after our vows of "till death do us part," the swollen nodes returned. In December when we were home for the holidays, I made a return visit to St. Jude. Again, the cowardly nodes withered under a professional's watchful eye. Dr. T. gave the same diagnosis. "Let's wait and see."

My parents were worried, too. Puzzled by the lack of action, they arranged for a private consult with another St. Jude doctor a few days later. Dr. S. had been one of my trusted St. Jude caretakers during and after my earlier treatment. This extended history instilled the confidence the younger Dr. T. had not yet earned.

Dr. S. recorded in the medical chart: *Told them we had no reason to suspect a recurrence—will discuss with Minda to determine how anxious she is. Mother and Minda have long-standing conflicts which are part of problem.*

(I cannot recollect any long-standing conflicts beyond the usual mother-daughter angst.)

1979, JANUARY

With no alteration in the game plan, we headed back to Nashville after the holidays. Over the next few months, the enlarged nodes hunkered down in their homey little spaces. They did not grow or shrink. Every few days I mustered up the courage to touch. No change meant a good night's rest.

Meanwhile, fatigue set in. Swollen nodes, fatigue, and worry—a foul combination. By spring, a persistent odor from the nodes became as bothersome as a decaying mouse lost in the bedroom air vents. But I was still being told not to worry. Easy for them to say. I crawled into bed every night thinking about those critters invading my private parts. They did not feel like a part of me. The OLD became older as my fingers gravitated to the nodes almost every night.

After taking a few weeks off from the nightly obsession, my ritual resumed with a big deep breath followed by the count. One, two, three. My hand slid down to my right groin. *Holy shit. They feel like they've grown again!* The largest one felt hard. Tender equaled good. Hard equaled bad. My worry meter shot up to the orange alert zone. GOSTRAIGHTTOTHEDOCTOR.

Screw St. Jude. I called Vanderbilt the next day and scheduled an appointment with Dr. Flexner. I was learning the art of waiting and worrying. When the background noise of worrying gets too loud or too frequent, it's time to check in with the experts.

Dr. Flexner, the benevolent commandant, delivered his opinions with a firm and resonating voice that was part of his larger-than-life presence in the Vanderbilt medical community. You did not ignore his advice. He demanded a biopsy right away. I welcomed the no-nonsense instruction to actually *do something*—a much-needed relief to resolve the mystery and move beyond the unrest. Barry and I had been hanging onto the edge for almost a year, and fatigue and worry were wearing my body and spirit down.

I checked into the outpatient surgery clinic for a biopsy of the node. Local anesthesia allowed conversation with the young surgeon as he prepped the site. "I see a lot of these nodes, and these lymph nodes are not cancerous. I can tell by the way they feel. And I'm almost always right," he boasted.

He was so confident in his batting average that I easily became a believer. After all, the St. Jude docs had the same hunch. Who was I to doubt these professionals? I went back to work the next day with the noose loosened around my long-constricted mood.

Barry's brother Danny and I were in the middle of the production of a training film for public health nurses called *The Road to Life*, showing how to accurately weigh and measure young children. That afternoon, the two of us, along with the rest of the production staff, finished a difficult scene at a local school. We had struggled for hours to simulate a bell-shaped curve by lining up—and keeping still—a group of elementary-aged kids. It was Friday. We were exhausted, so we headed to Carmen's for dinner and beer.

While the others were seated, I hurried to the pay phone hanging on the wall outside the restroom to call the doctor for the biopsy results. Dr. Flexner came right to the phone.

"We just got the pathology report. It was positive. The Hodgkin's disease is back. I'm so sorry, Minda. I wish I had better news."

I stood there in silence for a few moments. I wasn't really shocked. I had carried the suspicion with me for months, and although I'd suppressed the worry with positive feedback from Barry and the doctors, the fear had never ventured far away.

"It's not your fault. What's next?"

"Come in Monday morning, and we'll talk about it. We'll need to start chemotherapy as soon as possible."

I hung the phone on the hook and stood there staring at it for a very long minute. The verdict had an odd impact, as though I'd just received a potion of Valium laced with LSD. I was released from the purgatory of the unknown, but already dreading the thought of chemo running through my veins.

I dialed my parents' number. Then, as now, I needed the emotional lifeline to my mother and father. Dad answered the phone.

"Hi, Dad." My shoulders tensed as I strained to keep my composure. "I have not so good news. I have Hodgkin's disease again."

"Oh, nooo, Minda. Not again." There was a painful pause. In his undemonstrative, yet loving way, Dad communicated the same lack of surprise and worry. He was my hero in dealing with the demands of a corrupted body. He had twenty years of experience in quiet defiance, having lived with a crippling case of rheumatoid arthritis.

Our hearts and minds were on the same page. What a bummer. Oh, well. *Que sera sera.* Underlying this almost flippant reaction was confidence in the medical system. Finally, my year-old visitor's name and purpose were revealed, and something would be done to reverse its direction. *No action* had led me to fear that whatever "it" was would take control until it was too late to launch a successful attack. Now, no action was no longer an option.

As I hung up, I let out a relieving sigh and a few tears. Walking from the pay phone, I managed to gather myself to rejoin the group now celebrating the week's video shooting with beers in hand.

I slid into my seat and quickly unloaded, "I've got cancer again." Pause. "But I'm going to be okay." I grabbed the mug of beer waiting for me on the table and took a huge swig. They looked stunned. I changed the subject and did not mention it again. Being the men that men usually are, they didn't say anything about the emotionally laden news.

Over the weekend, a fissure split open in my rock-solid, eight-and-one-half-year relationship with St. Jude. Anger seeped up from the fracture like red-hot lava, and most of it was directed at Dr. T., not the institution. I had trusted her, and she had done me wrong. In retrospect, I see that I failed to bestow the respect and appreciation she deserved for avoiding another invasive procedure in light of the conflicting evidence.

The delay in uncovering the truth also gave birth to a broader, thorny-edged attitude toward "The Medical System" as a whole. I was particularly sensitive to the medical lexicon which can mislead and confuse patients. *Cured* was a term commonly cited by doctors to their cancer patients who survived five years without evidence of disease. Humbug. Here I was coming within reach of year nine, and the cancer was back. I felt betrayed by a medical establishment who had convinced me of one future, while knowing there is no such thing as a cure. Cure implies never again. Yet once you've had cancer, you are always at risk. Even if the risk goes down as the calendar moves forward, the body has shown a propensity toward letting abnormal cell growth go unchecked.

Yep, I was one angry gal, hurling my venom at a personified word that had grown fangs—*cured*—and at a cautious and compassionate St. Jude physician who, in my mind, at that time, wore a dunce's cap.

Where was an angry bitch to turn? Away from St. Jude and toward a local institution, Vanderbilt University Medical Center, where possibilities for a fresh pool of confidence awaited. I called St. Jude to share the new diagnosis and explain where I would be treated. Though I said I would visit St. Jude soon, I did not walk through those doors again for another sixteen years.

On Monday, Barry and I met Dr. Flexner for the second time. He was my kind of guy. Standing about five feet nine inches, with bright brown eyes, a welcoming smile, and just a touch on the well-fed side of life, he burst into the room much like Kramer would years later on *Seinfeld*. He was loud. He was bold. He was self-assured. No ifs, ands, or buts. Either you liked him or you didn't. There was no middle ground with a saucy persona like Dr. Flexner.

"Here's what we're going to do. Six months of chemotherapy. Two treatments every month. Two weeks on, two weeks off. If all goes well, you'll be done by December. The regimen of drugs we use now is called MOPP for the four drugs we'll give you. Nitrogen **m**ustard and vincristine [**O**ncovin] intravenously, and **p**rednisone and **p**rocarbazine by mouth for ten days after each treatment."

He stood there in his white coat, staring at Barry and me as if he had just given us his mother's favorite recipe for meatloaf. "Your chances for licking it this time are very good. We've treated lots of people since you had Hodgkin's years ago, and we know this formula works pretty well. Any questions?"

I shrugged. The plan was clear. I could only say, "All right. Let's just get on with it."

It sounded like the experimental treatment had progressed over the previous eight years from a nebulous guideline for dosage and duration to a well-defined formula. Both Barry and I were as ready as we were ever going to be. The first treatment was scheduled for Wednesday.

The Vanderbilt Medical Center, part of the Vanderbilt University campus, was a thirty-minute drive from our farm on Nashville's rural outskirts. On Wednesday morning, we loaded ourselves into the olive green '69 Valiant for the first of dozens of trips to and from what was to become another unforgiving hellhole. We parked a few blocks from the clinic and trekked through the 1920s residential neighborhood to my new medical home.

Over the previous few days, I had accepted the burden of another cancer sentence with eyes wide open to the havoc about to be imposed on my body. As I entered the clinic, a whirl of frantic memories bounced like Ping-Pong balls inside my head. My heavy feet moved me closer and closer to the haunting vision of white-coated drug pushers, needles, and vomit, aka the Torture Chamber.

The Vanderbilt clinics of 1979 were relatively low-budget operations with an interior motif similar to St. Jude's. Dingy chairs, dingy walls, dingy carpet. The only authentic source of brightness was Ms. Owens, the receptionist sitting behind the check-in counter. Her stunningly perfect smile and complexion and her calming good cheer greeted us each and every treatment day.

Just moments after settling into our seats in the waiting room, a nurse emerged to call us back to the Torture Chamber. The ingenuity of medical science had made a few improvements over the previous eight years, adding some comforting frills. This chamber was fully equipped to accommodate several victims, with an institutional version of a La-Z-Boy, a chair for the victim's hand holder, a rolling hospital cart, and a curtain which could be drawn all the way around the patient and hand holder to offer visual, though not audio, privacy.

Padded with pillows, the chairs were quite comfortable. Comfortable for the outside of my body, that is. Once I settled into position and the nurse took a few paces toward me with needles and vials of torture juice in hand, the inside of my body rebelled.

I doubt Pavlov was fully cognizant of how long-lived a reflex memory could be. Eight years separated me and the actual sensation of the cold, noxious liquid crawling through my veins. Yet *before* any physical contact between me and the needles for this first treatment, my heart hammered away, my throat tightened, and a queasiness already convulsed my stomach. When the nurse inserted the needle and the very first sensation of the cold chemo penetrated my arm, I began to heave. I was transported back to a time and place I had hoped to never revisit. Flashbacks. Oh, boy. Oh, boy.

It didn't take long to establish a routine. Barry and I took sick leave from our jobs on the day of each treatment. Outings to the Torture Chamber unfolded like this:

The alarm went off at 7:00 a.m. I consumed a hearty breakfast of a fried egg, whole wheat toast, and OJ so I would have something to eject. After breakfast, I changed into my chemo uniform, straight legged Levi blue jeans and a T-shirt. With Barry at the wheel of the Valiant, we drove into town and parked on Eighteenth Avenue. We walked four blocks to the clinic, usually in silence as I breathed deeply trying to take the edge off the anxiety.

I registered at the desk with Ms. Owens and headed down the hall for the obligatory blood drawing to confirm my body was still producing enough blood cells to tolerate the treatment. Then back to the clinic waiting area. Within a few minutes, my name was called. "Minda? How are you feeling?" the nurse inquired as she led us to an examining room.

"About the same," I replied, not in the mood for chitchat. I really wanted to tell her, *I feel like shit, worn out, bummed out, sun don't shine anymore in my neck of the woods. And you?*

A few minutes later, Dr. Flexner threw open the door and gave me the perfunctory physical examination with a check of my reflexes, my heart, my abdomen, and a finger feel of the nodes in my neck, underarms, and groin. The exam usually included a pleasant chat about my blood counts and how I was feeling. Occasionally we had an honest dialogue about my state of mind. At the end of the check-in, he gave me a prescription for the procarbazine, prednisone, and also Phenergan suppositories for nausea to be picked up on the way home.

We made our way to the Torture Chamber, and I settled into the chair with pillows and blankets. The nurse did what she could with what little she had to make me comfy. She then walked to the refrigerator wedged in the corner and pulled out two small vials of poison two to three inches in length. (I'm getting nauseated as I write this.) She walked toward me like a mad scientist, with a suspiciously awkward smile and needles and vials in hand. She performed this part of her thankless task rather nonchalantly, patient after patient, day after day, week after week, maintaining her armor against the misery she knew she was inflicting.

With her torture props expertly balanced in both hands, she pulled up a chair next to my side and sat down. I automatically stretched out my arm, knowing there was nowhere to run. She wrapped the fat, open-ended tourniquet around my upper arm just above my elbow and commanded, "Make a fist for me."

After flicking the inside of my elbow with her thumb and middle finger to get my veins to stand out, she inserted the IV needle into the juiciest, most rotund vein. Sometimes she hit the target right on the first time. Other times the veins were a bit obstinate, toughened up by the previous chemo treatments, so she would have to take another shot at finding a suitable port of entry.

"I'm in!" she would exclaim when she was successful. She then released the tourniquet and taped the needle into place. From the hospital cart, she grabbed the vial of faintly yellow, dishwater-like poison called nitrogen mustard. After snapping it onto the needle, she pulled back the syringe, drawing in a few drops of blood to make sure she had not disturbed the free-flowing connection to my bloodstream. Finally, she pushed the mustard ever so slowly into my vein.

It felt cold. The mustard was fresh out of the refrigerator, and as the cold sensation crept up my arm, spasms of nausea seeped upward from the pit of my stomach to the muscles of my throat. Up came my breakfast. A couple of minutes later, up came more breakfast. The last to emerge was a bitter, ironically mustard-colored bile. Then nothing. By this time, my GI tract was livid, and although there was nothing left in my stomach, the urge to vomit did not let up. So I heaved violently again.

In between my convulsions of vomiting, the nurse finished the mustard and inserted the smaller vial of poison number two, my old buddy vincristine. Exhausted from the GI revolt, I leaned back and entered a zombie state—awake with eyes partially opened, but withdrawn into my miserable little world. My breath was shallow, more like a tiny sniff. Each inhalation placed pressure on my stomach, resulting in a direct order to my brain to yell, "Vomit now!" So I lay as still as a feral cat in that moment before she leaps.

At some point in time, it was over. In a stupor, I stood up, gently swaying from side to side as I regained my center of gravity. Barry grabbed my hand, and we began to make our escape. I moved in *very* low gear, acutely aware of each muscle in my body propelling me forward, one step at a time. Moving too fast excited my GI tract. We walked out of the clinic, down the hall, and into the stagnant outdoors. It might have been fresh bracing air, but all I felt was inert oppression pushing in on me from all sides.

As we crossed Twenty-first Avenue away from Vandy's main campus, Barry lit up a joint. These were the days when, if you used discretion, you could smoke without fear. The pot smell alone cut through my altered state. He passed me the joint, and I smoked my way through the four blocks back to the car. On a vomit scale of one to ten, I left the clinic at eight, and the pot turned down my nausea to a two or three, which got me to the car without heaving. I crawled into the front bench seat of the Valiant, laid my head on Barry's lap, and drifted off.

Halfway home, we stopped at the Medicine Shoppe to pick up the prescriptions for the triple-*P* whammy of procarbazine, prednisone, and Phenergan. I snoozed restlessly while Barry went inside. At some point, I usually sat up, my head wobbling in a drug-induced fog. Invariably, this part of the trip home seemed to take hours. One time when I sat up suddenly, I found Barry staring at me through the pharmacy window. His tormented eyes pleaded with an unrestrained sadness he never let me see, as if to say, *How did we get here? This treatment is killing her.*

Barry returned to the car, drugs in hand. I lifted my head up slightly, enough to allow him to slide into the seat, and soon we were in the final stretch homeward. A few minutes later we turned onto our driveway, my head still in his lap. Without lifting my head, I knew where we were. The bumpy gravel driveway rattled my innards, but the relief of being minutes away from a soft mattress subdued my awakening GI tract.

Halfway down the mile-long driveway, I sat up and surveyed the passing pasture and woods. The sun was shining, but a surreal dimension lay between the brightness of the day and the dusk of my physical and emotional exhaustion—a place you reside when your spirit feels helpless. It doesn't seem quite authentic while you are there, yet you are keenly aware this limbo is your reality for a while. You know instinctively, like the heaviness in the air just before rain, that a torrent must fall to clear the sky. This is the space where I resided after each treatment.

When I stepped out of the car, Barry held my hand, and we waddled up the hill and the steps to our front door. With just a few more feet down the short hallway, alas, I was in our bedroom. I could not strip off my clothes fast enough. I tossed a nightgown over my head and sank into bed, heaving one last time for good measure. I inserted a Phenergan suppository and drifted off into a comatose sleep for hours, sometimes until the next day, even though it was barely afternoon.

When I awoke, my mood was somber, but my body pulled itself out of the bed, leaving the zombie shell behind in the tousled sheets. There was just a faint tinge of nausea in my gut. A cup of hot tea and mashed potatoes, lovingly prepared by Barry or my mother, slid down and soothed my shaken GI tract. Mmmmmmm. I shuffled back into the bedroom and into bed and quickly drifted off again.

The next time I opened my eyes, I was a new woman. Though still physically spent and emotionally flat, I was ready to make contact—with the natural outdoor world, not with people who expected something from me. A walk in the yard, through the garden, and down the driveway began flipping on the switches of my roughed-up mind and body. Contact with dirt, trees, growing vegetables, sunshine, and even rain peeled away the burly layer of funk shrouding my sense of aliveness.

Usually by day two or three, I was tuned up, ready for work and for contact with others beyond Barry. My administrative work took place at a desk, with pen and paper since there were no PCs yet. This allowed me to stretch out on a sleeping bag behind my desk when my body ran out of fuel. An hour's nap did the trick. Thank goodness for a sick-friendly workplace. After all, we *were* the Tennessee Department of Public Health.

Each day, I got stronger, gradually resuming normal activities—yoga, gardening, cooking, weaving, and socializing. And then it was time for the next CanceRid treatment. I hopped on the merry-go-round for another ride around the misery circle. With each subsequent assault, I went down faster and stayed down longer. The drugs had a cumulative impact similar to killing weeds with herbicides. The weeds might wilt and appear lifeless after the first treatment, but they sprang back. After more applications, though, the roots, stems, and leaves took longer to recover until at last the tormented plant withered.

After the first few treatments, Dr. Flexner cut the dose of vincristine in half to lessen my lethargy and the sensory nerve damage called neuropathy. Reminiscent of the battles from years earlier, the nerves in my hands and feet were in a tug-of-war with the vincristine, which caused tingling, numbness and involuntary cramping. Meanwhile, my red and white blood cells were fighting for their lives.

Two months after the diagnosis, I was woefully depressed, listless in body and spirit, frequently staring into space, and no fun to be with. On top of it all, a good friend battling his own demons had to go and kill himself. In an attempt to make sense of my despair, I developed a rudimentary theory of the origin of disease—where Jewish guilt meets Eastern philosophy.

MINDA'S THEORY OF THE
ORIGIN OF DISEASE
CIRCA 1979

GUILT
(From disappointing friends, mistreating Barry,
not resting enough, not eating enough whole grains,
not doing enough yoga, not meditating enough,
not managing stress well enough, not walking enough,
not being here and now enough.
Am I leaving anything out?)
↓
GUILT-ON-GUILT
(Guilt from feeling guilt—
as opposed to having guilt and blowing it off.)
↓
BLOCKED ENERGY CENTERS
(Or chakras—
the Eastern version of the heart and lungs
for the body's flow of energy.)
↓
IMPAIRED IMMUNE SYSTEM
↓
UNCHECKED GROWTH OF CANCER CELLS
↓
GRAND CONCLUSION:

GUILT = CANCER

Hence, unresolved emotions set the stage for the birth and growth of disease. I created the sources of the guilt; therefore, I caused the cancer. I was the Master of My Universe, in total control of this mess called my life. I was consumed with a long and growing list of Things I Done Wrong. I no longer viewed life in color. Rather, I saw the world in the gray shades of an East German town before the Wall came down.

Confounding this heavy case of the blues was a spiraling state of confusion and misgivings about the doctors and their methods. In my teens, I had possessed one hundred percent faith in the process. Now I found myself at the other end of the spectrum, totally doubting that these folks knew what in the hell they were doing. I felt like a bystander, observing the impact of the CanceRid on Mother Nature's primary defense, my white blood cells. These guys were supposed to protect me against intruders, yet the CanceRid was intentionally attacking them in a blatant case of friendly fire.

Relying on a mode of action that knowingly destroyed my body's natural defense seemed barbaric. Surely, the pool of knowledge that had propelled human beings through 239,000 miles of space to the moon could also concoct a drug that worked *cooperatively* with the body rather than *against* it. I felt aghast and disillusioned.

I faced two doors: Behind Door Number One lay the newest, 1979 version of traditional cancer treatment. Behind Door Number Two lurked some obscure alternative approach, and I was being forced to choose without a clear understanding of where either door might lead. Yet my life depended on it.

Time was not on my side. I felt compelled to choose quickly: *Will it be Door One or Door Two?* Two healing rays of sunshine helped light the way, yoga and meditation. Yoga classes and meditation instruction were opening up avenues to an entirely new way of thinking about the stimuli of disease and healing. My attraction toward Door Two was getting stronger and stronger.

Door Two offered a variety of maverick possibilities for self-healing, such as relaxation techniques and mental imagery. Fortunately, I had the advantage of a relatively sophisticated knowledge of the human body and disease. My undergraduate training in nutrition, with courses in physiology, microbiology, and biochemistry, generated a healthy dose of skepticism toward alternative medicine while nurturing a thin, but still functional confidence in evidenced-based scientific practices.

So I found myself in this suffocating room glaring at the two doors. The modern medicine behind Door Number One lacked intuitive appeal, but it had shown evidence of success. Door Number Two offered hundreds of years of alternative remedies and anecdotal wisdom – the true traditional medicine – but there was little scientific proof of its effect. I consulted my meditation teacher, Dr. Usharbudh Arya, who was traveling periodically to Nashville from his adopted home in Minneapolis to teach meditation to a bunch of young ignorant Americans.

"Take advantage of both," he told me.

With the tranquilizing voice of a gentle East Indian guru, he removed my dilemma. He challenged me to figure out ways to use relaxation, meditation, and other alternative practices to *help* the doctors and their chemotherapy do the job more effectively.

Robbie, my yoga teacher, gave me a cassette tape featuring Carl Simonton, an oncologist who explored the impact of mental imagery on the outcome of cancer treatment. I was spellbound by his story of a young boy with brain cancer. When all treatment options had been exhausted, Dr. Simonton assisted the boy in crafting his own mental imagery, visualizing the chemotherapy as a laser gun attacking his brain tumor. The boy was able to live out his fantasies of video war games in a real-life battle. The war was all in his head, and he had an endless supply of ammunition, so he kept the gun firing. He won his war—at least in the short term. (I have no idea if he is still alive.)

I listened to the tape again and again, feeling more and more empowered that I could take action to end my bystander role. Using visualization, I could now help my immune system support the CanceRid in doing its job. Modern and alternative forms of medicine were not mutually exclusive. Listening to the tape was just the impetus I needed to walk simultaneously through Door Number One *and* Door Number Two.

chapter five

1979, SUMMER

"Be here and be now. Remove yourself from all other places. Be aware only of the place in which you are sitting. Be here and be now."

As I repeated Dr. Arya's words, I sat cross-legged on the living room floor painting a mental image of my body healing itself. My goal was to replace the senseless rattling in my mind with a tangible connection to the inside of my body. Within a few minutes, I could feel and see the pale yellow chemo mingling in my blood, hitching a ride to the lymph nodes in my groin. The nodes vibrated as the killer juice seeped in and about the cells. One node at a time, I visualized the chemo burning up the cancerous cells from the inside out. I could feel the hot, sizzling sensation.

The impact of a chemo scalding was something I'd experienced first-hand. Once while receiving the CanceRid, the needle slipped out of my vein and infiltrated the tissue under my skin. It felt like a fire blazing inside my arm, and there was no way to reach in and snuff it out. "Getting under someone's skin" has had a personal meaning ever since.

After I had mentally attacked all the wayward cells I could "find," I scanned the nodes again. There's one more! *Zzzzzzt.* I moved to the next node, and the next, until I completed the reconnaissance. When my visualizations could no longer conjure up more mutant cells, a new image materialized. The chemo dripped around the nodes into all the nooks and crannies of my entire groin. It didn't make sense physiologically, but the imagery wanted to go there.

I opened my eyes. I felt relaxed, the edge was gone. A positive sense of well-being replaced the oppressive feeling that my guilt was aiding the enemy. I was not fully persuaded the imagery worked, but at that point, it didn't matter. I felt ninety-nine percent certain that replacing negative energy with positive vibes would boost my immune system.

Meanwhile, Barry was ready to resign as director of janitorial services for Minda's Department of Health and Misery. So far, he had received the highest marks on his performance, mopping up muck, changing sheets, doing and redoing laundry, enduring noxious smells, and using up all his sick leave from his day job. But he was exhausted. His vibrant partner in our back-to-nature lifestyle had been replaced by a pitiful, often bedridden, smelly vomit machine.

One regurgitated tuna sandwich finally pushed Barry over the edge. When he saw the brownish goop splattered across our white bedspread and oak hardwood floor, he threw up his hands and said, "You're on your own."

I couldn't blame him. Haggard and hung over from my last CanceRid cocktail, I slithered out of bed to strip the bedspread. I threw it into the washing machine and crawled back in bed, too spent to find another coverlet for warmth.

At these points of mounting stress, our need for a release valve became critical. Respite arrived in the form of my devoted parents. Mom and Dad drove in from Memphis and took over the cooking, cleaning, and nursing, allowing Barry to be Barry. They were the parents all children dream of, even tolerating the debauched pot smoking to help settle my tummy. But by late summer, more desperate intervention was needed.

A vacation on the beach!

During a two week break between treatments, Barry loaded my fragile body and our heavy backpacks onto a plane heading north. We were bound for Martha's Vineyard, but first, we stopped in Boston to visit Barry's Uncle Leo and his cousins Wilma and Gary, whom I had never met. Leo was a sommelier, a professional wine taster, and the oldest of my father-in-law's three surviving brothers. After a memorable stopover with wine-tasting, sailing, and finding common ground, our hosts took us to catch the ferry to the island.

I had been to Martha's Vineyard at the end of my freshman year with my college hall mate, Celia. She and I had masqueraded as two really hip chicks by taking her brother's MG to the island by car ferry. So as soon as Barry and I debarked at Oak Bluffs with our backpacks, we went in search of the funky Narragansett House where Celia and I had stayed. We didn't have far to walk. There she stood, a classic 1870s three-story

Victorian home as ramshackle and inviting as she had been a few years earlier.

Narragansett House was built for a captain and his lady. With a wraparound front porch on the first floor, two porches on the second, and a widow's watch on the third, the inn offered ample space to hang with your neighbors, which in this case were a bunch of scruffy baby boomers like ourselves.

One of our first adventures on the island was a trip to Zach's Beach, the nude bathing beach. In 1979, hitchhiking was an accepted mode of travel on this remote New England haven protected from the dangerous have-nots. After a short hike to the nearest highway outside the little town of Oak Bluff, we soon caught a ride to our destination. We had most of the beach to ourselves, with the exception of an elderly couple who obviously felt comfortable in their sagging one hundred percent natural attire. A time to dip, a time to swim laps, a time to bake, a time to stroll for shells, this was all part of an intentionally gradual healing time.

A walk to the other end of the beach led us to a grouping of boulders which had trapped a pool of muddy water several dozen yards from the tide's edge. A couple of young folk with still buoyant body parts had spread the mud from the pool over their entire bodies. We sat on the beach and waited patiently for our turn. Once alone, we went back to the pool and sank our feet into the mud. Next, we smeared each other head to toe with sandy muck, then stretched out on a boulder to bake. Warm sun hardened the mud like a layer of a chocolate coating a strawberry. We ran into the ocean to rinse off, then dried our cleansed skin in the sun for the final phase of our cancer spa treatment. I could not have found a more potent prescription for rejuvenation than this afternoon on the beach.

The next day we missed by just a few car lengths a social intercourse with one of the most famous residents of the island. After Barry and I met up on a beach with two fellow residents of the Narragansett House, the four of us wandered onto the road to hitch a ride back. Two people are more inviting to a passing car than four, so we split up.

"You two go first," the other couple kindly suggested, recognizing my limited stockpile of energy.

"No," I replied, as any bona fide southerner would. "I'm fine. You go on ahead."

The other couple walked several yards ahead of us to create some distance. Within a few minutes, a car pulled over to pick them up. A couple of cars later a Volkswagen Beetle pulled over for us. We climbed in the backseat and were delivered to the front door of the Narragansett House. Our housemates were waiting on the front porch plastered with two of the biggest smiles their sunburned faces would allow.

"You're not going to believe who picked us up!" the woman exclaimed. She was as excited as a little kid who had just returned from an unexpected visit to the ice cream parlor.

"Who was it?" Barry asked.

"James Taylor! Can you believe it? We caught a ride with James Taylor!"

Barry and I kicked ourselves for not cashing in on my disabled status to go first. The rest of our flings with free transportation were clumsy disappointments, and the kind drivers who transported us probably thought we were unappreciative. Little did they know we were expecting each driver to be James T. with his soulful, blue eyes and handsome hair—which he still had back then.

By the end of our stay on the island, I was healed. Hikes by the wild grapevines, moped rides to the beach, bicycle rides across the infamous Chappaquiddick bridge, laps and more laps in the ocean. The water, island sun, and adventures melted away the toxic leftovers of chemo and guilt. I landed on Martha's Vineyard down and out, dragging my feet. I left a few days later a few mental pounds lighter. Blue Cross Blue Shield, take note. A vacation to paradise could possibly be the most cost-effective measure for minimizing the effects of cancer treatment and expensive hospitalizations.

When our island cancer camp came to an end, we headed back to the mainland, rented a car and slowly meandered our way home via NYC and DC. We stopped in Virginia Beach for a visit to the Edgar Cayce Library. Cayce, considered by some as the father of holistic medicine, conducted hundreds of psychic "readings," guiding patients to improved physical and spiritual health. The library housed these readings and other recommendations of Cayce's for the diagnosis and treatment of various diseases.

Two days after our return, I resumed the CanceRid treatments, but unlike on previous treatment days, I skipped into the clinic with an upbeat attitude and a deceptively boundless reserve of stamina. The trip to

Martha's Vineyard had healed my broken spirit so that mainstreaming poison seemed tolerable, necessary, and doable.

My renewed zest was not powerful enough, however, to safeguard my still vulnerable GI tract. I recycled my breakfast during and after each treatment. Ass-kicking anti-nausea drugs were in order.

By 1979, the drug of choice to prevent nausea was Phenergan, delivered between the buttocks through a well-greased gelatin bullet. For us baby boomers with multiyear internships using mind-altering contraband, marijuana was another very effective companion. This weed thrived in the hot, humid summers of Nashville, so Barry and I stretched our gardening skills to avail my medicinal needs.

A couple of months after planting one small pot seedling in our vegetable garden, we found ourselves the proud parents of a four-foot plant. Then Mother Nature brought forth a torrential rain with high winds that snapped off the top third of the plant. For a while, we were angry at Mother N. because we assumed we'd have to obtain our medicinal herb the old-fashioned way—from resourceful friends with entrepreneurial leanings. To our amazement, Mother Nature's pruning, in combination with more frequent rains, transformed our little plant into a sturdy, seven-foot tree. Such a gift of bounty, blooming in my life as a savior, had to have a name. We christened her Big Bertha.

Given our paltry state salaries as public health officials, Big Bertha was a godsend. She calmed my GI tract again and again as the weeks of treatment wore on. THC was not yet available in pill form although research was underway, so we were allowed to use an examining room as our smoking parlor, though we didn't often use it. I never could get my mind around the vision of me and my bodyguard, Barry, exiting the examining room stoned, followed by a billow of aromatic smoke, while numerous pairs of bulging eyes gazed at us from the waiting room. I preferred to eject my breakfast *before* I left the clinic and then partake in the smoke-a-thon on our walk to the car.

Dr. Flexner was king of his castle, the Hematology Clinic. He had opinions about everything medical and otherwise, and nothing impeded his desire to share his viewpoint.

"I'm getting nauseous," I complained one day as he strolled through the Torture Chamber just as the nurse was pushing the plunger of mustard into my veins.

"You mean *nauseated*. *Nauseated*, not *nauseous*! You *make* me *nauseous*. I am *nauseated* around you. *Nauseous* is an adjective; *nauseated* is a verb. Remember that!" he barked in his fatherly style.

Phenergan plus pot plus the passage of time formed my bridge from stupor to consciousness. A few days after each CanceRid treatment, I began to venture into the city to hear music, see a movie, or walk the aisles of the grocery store. I was careful to stay within close proximity of a restroom just in case my GI tract got a little too active.

On one occasion, while visiting our parents in Memphis, my GI tract reminded me of who was in control. We had just enjoyed a family dinner at a Chinese restaurant, and as we were exiting through the double front doors, another couple approached the entrance. Their mouths must have been watering in response to the Chinese aromas swirling about.

"How's the food?" the man asked.

Without warning, I ejected my meal at his feet. I stared at the pool of churned shrimp lo mein, then looked up at the couple who were now glaring at me.

"I am so sorry," I said, too embarrassed to look them in the eye. I paused for a moment, not sure what explanation, if any, to offer. Then I added, "The food was actually delicious."

Barry headed inside to get help to clean up the mess.

By late September, with two more rounds of CanceRid to go, my body took a detour. I developed a nonproductive cough and a nighttime fever unresponsive to Tylenol. When my fever peaked at a virulent 103 degrees, two possible culprits were suspect: an infection gaining ground over my weakened immune system, or the cancer gaining ground over the chemo. Dr. Flexner sentenced me to the Vanderbilt inpatient unit to figure out what was going on.

With the proper spectacles, a hospital stay can be seen as an adventure. Adventure implies you are heading into unknown territory with a risk of danger and perhaps a dubious outcome. Yessiree, anytime you put your body in the care of a team of health care professionals with round-the-clock access to an unlimited amount of equipment, advice, and homeless microorganisms, an adventure is possible. Often, hospitals are absolutely vital to our survival when a bodily function goes awry. Paradoxically, they also can be places for many screw-ups and no clear answers.

After several months of treatment, my immune system was floundering. Unfortunately, the CanceRid was not smart enough to distinguish between the good guys and the bad guys. A lot of the good guys, my white blood cells, were unintended casualties. The high mortality rate of these foot soldiers of infection defense left my body scrambling for help to fight off menacing foreign organisms. The body needed a break from the onslaught until the white blood cells could get sufficient reinforcements.

Dr. Flexner's plan of attack was twofold: (1) help the good guys by pumping my body with high doses of broad-spectrum antibiotics to deluge bacteria of all different shapes and sizes, and (2) peruse the lymph system for signs of unchecked cancer. The antibiotics took hold rather quickly. Within a couple of days, my fever was down. All signs pointed to a bacterial infection.

When my blood work returned from the lab, the results showed my white and red blood cells had taken too big a hit from the last CanceRid treatment. Reinforcements were needed right away. I was hooked up for a transfusion of three units of packed red blood cells.

Meanwhile, Dr. Flexner began his hunt for other cancer cells. Bone marrow biopsy number three was ordered. Compared to the nightmarish procedure from years earlier, this biopsy was not nearly as painful. I'm not sure whether the needle or the needle handler was the source of such dramatic improvement. This test coupled with a CT scan revealed no obvious signs of new growth, but there was ambiguity in the results.

My confidence was not boosted when I overheard Dr. Flexner and a colleague debating about the appropriate course of action. Midway through a battle, one generally wants to hear a level of certainty from one's commander erring on the side of arrogance. Yet my two four-star generals didn't sound certain about anything. Although my skepticism of modern medicine had been growing, I had placed a sizeable quantity of emotional stock in my bright doctors and their well-defined recipe for success. We were to that point of salt to taste, however. To my uneducated ear, it seemed the generals were guessing and opted for a lot more salt.

At length, Dr. Flexner gave me the good and not so good news. Unaware I had listened in on their discussion, he presented the treatment schedule with his usual decisiveness. "We don't see any clear signs of disease, but four, instead of two, more rounds of chemotherapy will help diminish chances of further growth."

During the final few days of my hospital stay, a minor event reminded me of the potential risks when too many people have responsibility for dispensing health care to too many patients in one large institutional setting.

"Time for your birth control pills," said the nurse as she extended the little white pleated paper cup toward my face.

The absurdity of the error caught me off guard. "Uh, I don't think those are for me. I don't take birth control pills. I don't even have much of a period."

"The order is in your chart." Again, she thrust the cup toward my face.

"Chart or no chart, I'm not taking any birth control pills!" I was beginning to get impatient, and I pushed the cup away to fend off any further pressure from this drug pusher.

"Have it your way." She left and didn't return. It was never mentioned again.

Day ten of Minda's Hospital Adventures offered another challenge.

"Where is my wife?" Barry asked the attendant at the nurses' station. He had left work early to pick me up and take me home, but he'd found my room vacant.

"Well, let's see here."

The attendant floundered for a few minutes, tracking down the floor nurse assigned to my room, who didn't have a clue of my whereabouts. The staff talked among themselves, trying to summon up a reasonable explanation for the increasingly worried spouse. Another nurse walked up to the desk, overheard the discussion, and enlightened the puzzled staff.

"She was taken down to X-ray, but that was a couple of hours ago. She should have been back by now."

"Where is the X-ray department?" Barry asked. With directions in hand, he dashed out of the unit with a mission: *find Minda.* Wasn't that the hospital's job?

Ten minutes later, Barry found me sitting in a wheelchair in a busy thoroughfare. I was facing the wall looking as dejected as a kid in time-out. There was a simple explanation. They forgot about me.

I've since personally witnessed Vanderbilt Hospital staff working hard to improve their care, but this innocent oversight came at a particularly wrong time and place. The X-ray technician had completed her job, and unaware of my plummeting white blood cells, she had parked me in the hallway to be escorted back by the attendant. The attendant never showed.

As I sat in the wheelchair in the busy hallway, my anxiety about infection morphed into delusional paranoia. The stream of human traffic mutated into a swarm of infectious bugs, against whom I felt defenseless. Finally I turned my wheelchair to face the wall rather than see the dangerous crowd of passersby. I folded up the wheelchair footrests and nuzzled as close to the wall as possible. There I sat, believing the attendant would eventually show up. What a surprise when the attendant turned out to be Barry!

When we got back to the room, I was discharged with strict orders to be wary of infection and dark stools indicating possible loss of blood. My surviving platelets were hanging on for dear life, and my white blood cell count had dipped to a precariously low level. Dr. Flexner announced the chemo treatments were off until further notice. I was relieved to hear he was not releasing me from the shackles of this well-oiled medical machine into the healing arms of the Torture Chamber nurses. We went home for a reprieve from the CanceRid, and a few days later I returned to work, resuming an almost full routine of site visits and paper work to help monitor the quality of our health clinics.

Fortunately, the final weeks of treatment for the Hodgkin's relapse were unremarkable. This second war with the cancer demons drew to a close with the sixteenth treatment in November, 1979, six months after the diagnosis. As Barry and I walked toward the '69 Valiant, I inhaled shallow, palliative puffs of cannabis. This time around, the stroll was more of a strut. I was in charge now, not the doctors, not my GI tract, not my lymph nodes. The zombie persona was still dominant, but I was able to view the gray surroundings with a backdrop of sunshine rich with the autumn remnants of oranges, reds, and greens. Even the browns had depth. My canvas was quickly coming alive.

Once again, in a relatively short period, I had filled another large file with solemn memories. And once again, the mental and physical wounds were more of a blessing than a curse. I walked away with daily reminders of the value of listening to your inner voice and reacting before it is too late. I'd gained a fresh view on what my roles in health and disease could and should be. At age twenty-four, I felt triumphant, trusting in my ability to be an active player in maintaining a robust life with or without cancer. But the true value of these experiences was yet to be revealed.

chapter six

1980

Cancer comes at you fast. One minute you are waltzing through life worrying about whether to switch your dog to low-cal dog food; the next minute you are emerging from the doctor's office with your life—every part of your being—whitewashed with mind-bending questions. What doctor should I use? Should I seek a second opinion? From whom? Should I pursue chemo? Do I need radiation? Do I have to do any of this at all? What happened to yesterday?

It's no wonder that in the midst of juggling all these details, life *after* cancer treatment rarely enters the discussions. The long-term impacts on your well-being seem insignificant when you are plotting a course that keeps you alive for as long as possible. At the end of the course, you are eager to move on and leave the details behind.

Then one day, having moved on with life as you knew it in the BC (before cancer) years, you are sitting at your desk at work contemplating how to squeeze one more stop at the grocery into your schedule. Without warning, a peculiar sensation darts through your chest. What was that?

Welcome to the Cold War era of your cancer conflict.

In January, 1980, within a month after my last CanceRid treatment, I was naïvely wallowing in the afterglow of victory when the lingering effects of the treatment began to appear. Hypogonadism, cervical dysplasia, herpes zoster (shingles), infertility, skin cancers, a collapsed lung—a cascade of problems materialized as my Cold War years got under way.

While in the dreamless void of a comatosely restful sleep, I was shaken into consciousness by a pulsating, fire-engine red sting of heat. A creepy tingling led to profuse unfeminine sweating as the heat enflamed my face, neck, scalp, arms, legs, and even the bottoms of my feet. Still in my twenties, I was not yet thinking about hot flashes. And yet, in what seemed like a nanosecond, I had mutated into the sweat hog from hell. With one swift move, I grabbed the sheet and blanket and threw them onto the floor.

"What the hell is wrong with you?" Barry sat up in bed, the look on his face telling me I better have a good answer.

"Let's have sex?" I asked, the only response I could think of that would change his grimace to a smile even if the house was on fire.

I continued before he could answer. "Actually, I was sound asleep when I suddenly started sweating as if I'd just made a mad dash up the hill. I'm soaked. I'm going to take a shower."

I got out of bed, took a shower, and changed into a fresh, clean gown. Barry went back to sleep. So did I. With the clamminess gone, I slipped back into the coma-like sleep that post-chemo patients crave.

A consultation with Dr. Flexner unveiled the first of many secrets about the collateral damage my treatment had inflicted. My ovaries had taken a hard hit from the chemo and were befuddled about their mission. They no longer pumped out enough estrogen to help regulate my thermostat. The result? Hot flashes. Learn to live with them.

The dwindling supply of estrogen also explained why my periods were light and sporadic. Ovarian failure, as the condition is formally known, spawned erratic mood changes. Sometimes, I was a peaceable, PMS-less persona, and other times, my body was on fire with hot flashes and unfounded rage. My ovarian cells no longer had control over the intensity or regularity of their cycles.

Despite recommendations to start estrogen supplements to keep the hot flashes at bay, I chose to let Mother Nature run the show. College courses in endocrinology and biochemistry had taught me about the diffuse power of hormones, and a little voice whispered, *It's not nice to fool Mother Nature.* Hormones were one of the Mother's workhorses, causing effects far beyond the visible. Using these babies without full knowledge of the potential fallout could be as dangerous as grabbing Dumbledore's wand and waving it indiscriminately. So I said, "Thanks, Dr. Flexner, but I'll pass and endure the hot flashes for now."

Each of my body parts reacted in their own way to messages from their chemo-stymied cells, and in month two of the post-CanceRid era, my cervix had her turn in the spotlight. In contrast to my emaciated ovaries, the cervix became too spunky. Precancerous dysplasia cells, not unusual in young, sexually active women, promptly multiplied, progressing from moderate to severe in a few short months. Amid these cells was a growth on my cervix, or lesion as the doctor called it, about the size of a small date.

The advisable thing to do, according to the mild-mannered, soft-spoken Vandy gynecologist, Dr. B., was to hack away with a knife, removing a conical-shaped section of my cervix. Dr. Jekyll and Mr. Hyde come to mind when I envision the gentle, dedicated Dr. B. using saws, knives, and potent radiation beams to heal. I asked him for a reprieve before undergoing the knife again. I did not tell Dr. B., but I hoped a couple of weeks might buy me time to apply mental imagery to the damaged tissue.

I set to work with a daily practice, imagining the slow, timely destruction of the unwanted tissue. Each morning, I sat crossed-legged on my sky blue zafu meditation pillow. In my mind's eye, I used a toothbrush with densely clustered wire bristles and a very short handle to gently scrub the brown, semi-stiff, thumb-shaped growth on all sides. I could hear the bristles making contact. Day after day, for fourteen days, I whittled away, watching it get smaller each day. I could feel it resisting, yet withering under the friction of the brush, though it never disappeared.

When I checked into the hospital, my attitude was resoundingly positive. I had done my part to quell my fears and negativity. To avoid the fogginess in the after-surgical hours, I made a special request for a spinal block to deaden the pain instead of the general anesthesia. Consequently, I was awake during the surgery. Shivering uncontrollably from the frigid temperatures of the operating room and regretting my decision about anesthesia, I heard Dr. B. tell the anesthesiologist how surprised he was that the lesion had shrunk from just two weeks ago! A tiny smile slipped through my rigid grimace and chattering jaws.

After the surgery, the tech rolled me on a gurney to a hospital room. There was no need to linger in a recovery room for the awakening from the general anesthesia. Having never felt so alert after surgery, I was ready to get up and move. I walked up and down the hall several times, excited by the outcome of the surgery and my clarity. Bad idea. Very bad idea. I walked back to my room and fell asleep. When I woke up from the nap, I had the most excruciating headache I had ever experienced. Just lifting my head a couple of inches sent this agonizing pain pulsating through the entire circumference of my skull. The pain ceased when I lowered my head all the way down directly onto the mattress.

I called the nurse, the nurse called the doctor, and in walked an anesthesiology resident. "You shouldn't have gotten up after the surgery. Didn't someone tell you the spinal fluid could leak out of the puncture wound from the block?"

His scolding made me feel like a naughty patient, but unfortunately, no one had informed me of a cardinal rule for spinal blocks: *do not stand up for at least eight hours in order to allow the puncture in the spine to heal.* Now the only remedy was to lie perfectly flat until the fluid regenerated and the wound healed.

I was discharged the next day with a prescription for complete bed rest. So much for the quicker healing time with a spinal block. A couple of days later, the agonizing drumbeat was still activated by lifting my head. My favorite uncle, an anesthesiologist in LA, called to see how I was doing. When I explained my predicament, Uncle Stanley suggested a quick solution.

"I can call in a prescription for Dexedrine. I don't know why, but we've found it works really well for the pain of a headache from a spinal fluid leak."

Barry picked up the prescription on his way home from work. One dose of Dexedrine and the headache vanished. I was up and about that evening and back to work the very next day. My devoted Uncle Stanley had always been my favorite uncle, but now he topped the list of all my relatives. In a matter of hours, I went from an immobilized slug to a worker bee with a Type-A drive, ready to take on the world. (Yes, this wonder drug was the same diet pill that was peddled for all-nighters in college, though I can proudly confess I succumbed to the study aid only once.)

A few months passed before the next Cold War event. A benign-looking rash developed on my back. At that time, a good friend from Memphis named Felix was visiting for the weekend. He was a second-year medical school student, so I said, "Hey, I've got this funny-looking rash on my back. Want to see it?"

Felix was eager to share his hard-earned, but questionable expertise, so I pulled up the back of my shirt and showed him the crop of small red welts. They looked like a bad case of poison ivy, covering an area the size of a mango on the right side of my back. The rash was smarting me with sharp prickles edging toward three on the one-to-ten pain scale, ten being the most painful.

"Shingles. I'm sure of it. We just studied this last week in neurology class." Felix was so pleased he could give an educated opinion. As much as I loved my dear friend, though, I could not summon up much faith in the diagnosis of a second-year medical student.

Straight out of *War of the Worlds*, the 2005 Hollywood film where the alien invader spreads its tentacles across the suburban lawn, my red colony blossomed as the weekend wore on until they reached the edge of my back and turned the corner toward my rib cage. The invader was held at bay by the continental divide of my nervous system, limiting the infection to the right side only. Meanwhile, the oldest spots expanded into dime-sized blisters running together like mountain ranges. The pain climbed to a six as my electric current fired out of control. These lightning bolts, although brief, grew more and more frequent, and Felix encouraged me to go to the emergency room, forcing us to cancel a planned backpacking trip.

The Vandy ER physician, with no more than three years up on Felix, stared in awe at my body sculpture. "Herpes zoster," he said without missing a beat. "Also called shingles." He did not have to leave the room to consult a book or the attending physician. Bingo, Felix! I was so impressed with my learned friend.

"I've never seen a full-blown case like this," the ER physician marveled. He explained in detail about the nature of herpes zoster and where "we" might go from here.

Pardon the digression here for a few words while I unload. Physicians often say "we," like husbands often refer to "our" pregnancy. In this instance, I found the usage offensive. After all, I was making the sacrifices 24/7, and although the doc was a key player, I wanted all the credit I could get. Now back to "our" rash.

Herpes Zoster and Herpes Varicella are the two-headed Siamese twins commonly known as shingles and chicken pox, respectively. Varicella is the meeker sister. She prefers to keep company with young children. Zoster takes the backseat for many years until one day she decides to push her humble sister out of the way. You see, Zoster has a more abusive personality with an affinity for hosts who are down on their luck, such as the elderly or anyone with a weakened immune system. Zoster preys on defenseless cancer patients who've been doused by immune-suppressing chemo. My body was still recovering from the multiple doses of CanceRid when Zoster took control.

I learned from the doctors that the Herpes twins probably found a port of entry into my body when I contracted a simple case of chicken pox as a child. Varicella didn't demand too much attention, and I wasn't even aware that she and her evil sister were still hanging around. Zoster was lurking, though, wide awake and waiting for an opportune moment for her coming out party. Now she was firing away, wearing out the sensory nerves in the right side of my chest.

"Fortunately, we have a new antiviral drug," the ER doctor explained. "It's called acyclovir, and in your case, it should be given intravenously." He was young, but he had no doubt in his voice. "We're going to admit you to the hospital so we can observe the rash and make sure we're getting the shingles under control."

So began Hospitalization Number Six. Before I knew it, Varicella woke up from all the racket and did not want to be left out. To stop her overbearing sister from stealing the limelight, she spread tiny pink chicken pox bumps all over my skull, gradually creeping closer to my right eye. Zoster and Varicella bonded as they never had before, and the doctors went to work to calm these girls down.

Over the next several days, a parade of Vanderbilt interns, residents, and hematology and oncology fellows paraded through my hospital room to gawk at the growing mass of blisters. My case offered a unique opportunity to see the new drug in action, and I was glad to oblige.

"Come on in," I replied to Dr. Flexner as he entered my hospital room with four students in tow. *Sure,* I thought, *I don't mind if five grown men gather around my bed and glare at my bare chest.*

The truth was, I did not mind. I was well indoctrinated by the previous St. Jude and Vanderbilt experiences into the gallant role of the medical model. It felt as natural to me as smiling for a family photo. I could sometimes feel the uneasiness of some of the younger medical students, however, because their eyes failed to meet mine. Several of the onlookers said it was the biggest clump of Zoster lesions they had ever seen. My body was no slacker when it came to growing things.

As the days wore on, the blisters blew their tops like little volcanoes, oozing their contents until they started to scab over. The pain diminished, and my head stopped itching. Acyclovir worked. On day nine, I was discharged. My miniature mountain range of blisters had become an assortment of flattened stumps colored pale walnut to burnt cedar.

Nearly thirty years later, I still have the party favor Zoster left behind. In addition to the scars, shielded from vision just under the skin is a network of damaged nerves that still tingle at times. Zoster installed a switch, set to kick on when the weather becomes frigid. Indoors or out, the damaged nerves start firing and itching whenever I get chilled. Scratching won't appease the itch; the source of the irritation is too deep for the penetration of my nails. So I breathe deeply, rub firmly, cover myself up, and it usually subsides.

1982

No bombs went off over the next couple of years, and on July 15, 1982, I woke up, opened my eyes, and savored the triumph of reaching my twenty-eighth year of life. I assumed a Johnny Carson-style smirk on my face, smug and understated. Hot diggity dog. I made it! Little Miss Fortune Teller, who'd predicted my early demise at the age of twenty-seven, was now an authenticated charlatan. My smile lingered for days as the psychological shackles of her spell broke apart once and for all.

I had long feared that heavy stress might bring back the cancer demons, but two months after my birthday, I took a bold step to face that fear. I entered graduate school. I enrolled at the University of Tennessee in Knoxville to pursue a master's degree in nutrition science, a probable mother lode of stress. For the previous five years, I had intentionally kept my life calm, with a low stress job and extracurricular interests I could always cancel if I got scared. Now I was ready to see if I could undertake stress-inducing goals while maintaining good health with plenty of sleep, yoga, exercise, and wholesome food.

Barry and I rented our house to our friend Jimmy and took up residence in a funky log cabin on the edge of Knoxville belonging to my major professor. The cabin was constructed like a *Ripley's Believe It or Not* Museum. Depending on where you stood in the kitchen, the steeply slanted ceiling made you feel like either a lanky giant with just four inches of headroom or a squatty gnome with several feet of empty space overhead.

In the small crooked cabin, I developed a textbook case of menopausal symptoms—frequent hot flashes, violent mood swings, droopy breasts, drying and loosening skin, and irregularity in timing and flow of menstrual cycles. Once again, no one had forewarned me of this possibility. Holding fast to the belief of total control, I had filed away the earlier bout of hot flashes. But now, as these new hot flashes increased in frequency to eight or ten per hour, I became accustomed to looking and feeling like I had just returned from picking cotton in the back forty.

There was no use in showering during the day; the next sweat fest was never far behind. So I looked forward to the few moments after my evening shower when my skin was not sticky and clammy. If I was lucky, I would have time to get dressed after emerging from the shower before the next flash hit.

During one forty-eight-hour spell, I morphed into a schizophrenic witch who refused to leave her bed. I lay there laughing at Barry's quick-witted retorts one minute, and sixty seconds later, I rained tears of despair. Laughing, crying, laughing, crying, I curled up under the covers on Friday evening and emerged from my cocoon only for bathroom and mealtime breaks.

On Sunday evening, the mood swings passed as quickly as they had surfaced. I thought, *What in the hell is wrong with me?* Maybe the pressure of Dr. Smith's bioenergetics course was pushing me over the edge, presenting more stress than my challenged body and brain could handle.

I headed to Nashville to consult my gynecologist and my new hematologist, Dr. Seth Cooper. I had tired of Dr. Flexner's abrupt bedside deportment. Dr. Cooper proffered a gentler disposition better matched to the needs of the maintenance phase I had entered. After talking with these two physicians, I had much more information than I was prepared to receive.

Both doctors informed me no children were in my future—at least the kind that had my genes. The stark message landed in my lap like a grenade. The prognosis was confirmed by a third doctor, a fertility specialist. All three doctors recommended a panacea for the hot flashes, supplemental estrogen and progesterone, commonly known as hormone replacement therapy, or HRT. Despite the seemingly innocuous and essential-sounding "replacement therapy," I opted to reject the prevailing wisdom. My telepathic gut communicated loudly once again, *Beware of those powerful hormones*.

Each doctor gave the same dramatic prognosis. "Your ovaries have entered a phase of no turning back."

My chronologically young, but physiologically aged ovaries were producing sporadic dribbles of estrogen instead of a well-controlled, flowing faucet of the stuff. In the intricate feedback system of hormones, where one hormone-producing organ depends on another for the signal to adjust the spigot, my ovaries were left in the lurch. As a result, another reproductive hormone, FSH, was skyrocketing out of control. (Stick with me here if there is interest in the inner workings of fertility or the onset of menopause. Otherwise, leap forward four paragraphs.)

FSH, or follicle-stimulating hormone, together with LH, luteinizing hormone, are released from the pituitary gland for one purpose—to stimulate one follicle in the ovary to spit out one egg one time per month. (Mother Nature is not perfect. On occasion more than one egg or follicle gets stimulated.) When the FSH and LH reach a very specific level, an egg bursts forth from the mature follicle and hightails it to the neighboring fallopian tubes and then down into the uterus where she can be fertilized by one of the incoming sperm.

Just prior to the emergence of the egg, called ovulation, the FSH level starts to drop. It continues to drop in the days after ovulation, and this lower level of FSH is the green light for *increasing* the secretion of estrogen. This gradual rise in estrogen and its comrade progesterone after ovulation is essential to help the uterus get nice and comfy for the fertilized egg. If the egg remains single, or the now bonded egg and sperm fail to take up residence in the uterus, the estrogen and progesterone drop, causing the uterus to rid herself of the excess baggage. She sloughs away the unneeded vascular padding, and this weeping of the welcome mat for the fertilized egg is better known as menstruation. Next, a very delicate dance among the levels of each of the hormones results in the cycle beginning again.

So, FSH needs estrogen, and estrogen needs FSH. Without the stability and support of each other at the right time, they get thrown off course. A prolonged deficiency in estrogen, as with post-chemo trauma or advancing age, leads to levels of FSH that climb higher and higher – eventually into the land of the barren.

When the rising levels of FSH dash off the chart, the doctor concludes estrogen is in short supply. No estrogen, no babies. No estrogen, no thermostat control. On the positive side, no estrogen, no UMS (ugly mood swings).

All three physicians bore the same definitive, disheartening news. "When the FSH levels go up as high as yours, we rarely, if ever, see it drop low enough again to support a pregnancy."

In an instant, I felt an overwhelming desire to have children. Prior to the news of my infertility, I had a vague longing for offspring, but it was not imprinted on my To Do list as vividly as college and career, country living and gardening, yoga and meditation, weaving and photography. But the jolting news about my inability to procreate changed a dim desire into an insatiable lust. I must have a child. *Now!*

Imagine this. I'm lying on my back in bed in the dark, just having made love with Barry. The sheets are tangled, nightgown on the floor. Barry has gone to the kitchen. My buttocks are elevated a few inches off the mattress by a pillow, and my legs are fully extended into the air at a ninety-degree angle to my belly. While I am in this modified yogic shoulder stand, my eyes are closed as I envision the sperm swimming as fast as they can up my vagina, through the cervical canal and up next to the uterine wall where the lone sexy egg is waiting.

The spermies have bright eyes and wide grins on their faces as their tails are flittering as fast as hummingbird wings, racing to be the winner of this once-in-a-lifetime contest. One sperm picks up speed and leaves the rest of the contestants behind. As he gets closer to *her*, he changes from a shade of gray to bright red. Bam! He crashes headfirst into Miss Egg. In my mind, there is an explosion of red, orange, and yellow as the egg and sperm become one. Then I open my eyes and get up to join Barry in the kitchen for a bowl of Mayfield's chocolate ice cream.

And so it went for over a year. I stuck to the regimen like a religious fanatic. Month after month. Explosion after explosion. I began to lose hope, but kept to the ritual anyway, until the quest for fertility eventually slipped down my To Do list and was replaced by the quest for completing my thesis and graduating.

1984

One perfect morning of May, 1984, I sat at my desk in the cabin working on my thesis while I munched away at a stack of saltine crackers. Allergies always made me nauseous (oops—nauseated). I was staring out the window, saltine in hand, pondering whether to add another table of statistics to my thesis when another quandary crept into my head as softly as a gentle breeze and nudged the thesis aside. This nausea was clearly different from the queasiness of allergies. Spring was not the time of year I experienced problems with allergies. The leaves of fall were the usual culprit. So what was making me nauseated?

Holy moly! I'm pregnant!!!!!!!!

I leaped from my rickety chair in the rickety sunroom of the rickety cabin and dashed outside to my car. The closest drugstore was less than a mile away. As I drove to the store, I envisioned my baby zygote pulsating with life, burrowing comfortably into my uterus. The excursion to and from the store passed so quickly, it seemed practically nonexistent. I got home, ripped open the box containing the pregnancy test, and gingerly conducted the experiment.

Blue for yes! The test strip was a beautiful deep purple-blue. Praise the Lord! I danced in circles as I felt the fertility gods hovering over me. Then I dashed back to the car and headed for Barry's office. Waves of euphoria propelled me toward him like the sperm toward the egg. I pulled into the parking lot of his office, bolted out of the car, bounced up the steps of the Regional Health Department two at a time, swung open the front door, and raced toward Barry's cubicle.

"Guess what?" In the typically submissive character that becomes me, I did not give him time to answer. "I'm pregnant!"

Barry was in such disbelief, afraid to believe, all he could say was, "How do you know? Are you sure?"

"Well, I'm pretty damn sure!" I convinced him of the evidence, although he remained a tad cautious until the visit to the gynecologist confirmed the results.

After I completed my thesis and oral exam for the master's degree, we moved back to Nashville for the final trimester. An arrogant, right-to-new-life attitude carried me through both the pregnancy and the delivery as I naïvely deduced that I had paid my medical dues and was entitled to a healthy nine-month pregnancy culminating in a healthy progeny. I got just what the patient ordered.

1985

On February 2, 1985, a heavy snowstorm was forecast, so Barry and I slept in the city at Eric and Fran's house, just in case or our mile-long driveway and the roads into town might be covered with a foot of snow. Just after midnight, I got up to go to the bathroom, and as I leaned over the toilet, out gushed a lot of water. It was my first time around, but the volume was obviously more than my bladder usually released. I cleaned myself up and got back into bed, hesitant to set the wheels into motion. I was reluctant to wake my snoring birth assistant, who was exhausted from a full day of urban cross-country skiing.

Then I felt the first labor pain. I tapped Barry's shoulder lightly. "Psst. Psst. Barry, wake up."

No response. He was in a deep sleep. Hours of aerobic exercise, exposure to the winter elements, and a couple of Budweiser Tall Boys had mellowed this father-to-be.

I shook him harder. "Wake up, Barry. *Wake up*!"

"What?" he replied with a hint of annoyance at being yanked out of his much-needed sleep.

"I think it's time. My water broke."

"Can't it wait until morning?" His attempt to lighten the gravity of the moment did not work.

"No!"

Daddy jolted into action. I was always amazed at his ability to cross the barrier from a REM sleep state to full alertness. After waking up Fran and Eric for moral support, I called Dr. Barnett, my obstetrician (not Dr. B., the gynecologist from years earlier). A description of my now increasing labor pains resulted in the high sign to head to the hospital. Barry called my other two labor assistants, my best friend Ava and Barry's brother Danny, who was the designated photographer.

We drove slowly through the dark, deserted, snow-covered streets and were admitted to the birthing suite. As the labor contractions cycled, my able assistants sat on the sofa a few yards away enjoying a Jungle Jim movie. During commercials, or if I let out a particularly inhuman call of distress, they swung into action, holding a hand, guiding my breathing, massaging a leg, or snapping a photograph. Actually, my three assistants along with Dr. Barnett and the labor nurse did everything right, helping when needed and keeping their distance when not.

Six hours after admission, at 7:32 a.m., our miracle child was born in the most spiritually moving event Barry and I had ever experienced. Our baby girl weighed in at seven pounds, ten ounces with a APGAR score signifying rosy good health. We named her Shea, the child who wasn't meant to be.

For a few months, my body and I made peace. Shea and I reveled in our mother-daughter bonding, breastfeeding, and resting. Shea was a gentle, easy-to-please baby.

When Shea was five months old, the Cold War resumed. She and I were resting on the living room sofa when I felt an itch under my left arm, just at the lower edge of my armpit. A serious attempt to scratch the alleged chigger bite revealed a flesh-colored tab of protruding skin. The tiny appendage looked so alone, as if all the skin covering my breast had been tucked into my bra, with this one forlorn piece inadvertently left behind. Because of the irritating location, I made an appointment with a dermatologist to have it removed.

Dr. P. clipped off the little outsider. Barely a drop of blood was sacrificed, as if the tab were glued on and not actually part of me. The visit was quick, the procedure painless, and the prognosis reassuring. A few days later, I received a letter from Dr. P. In one sentence, void of any emotion, I was informed I had basal cell carcinoma.

Please call if you have any questions, the letter advised.

If Dr. P. had been in my presence, I would have spewed every unkind, foul-mouthed word this sheltered young woman could conjure up, which at the time was not much. Today, I would have much more graphic ammunition in my stockpile. I had never heard of basal cell cancer. UV rays, 10:00 to 2:00 sun, and signs of skin cancer were not yet included in the common vernacular of cancer risk discussions. In my chemo-weary mind, hearing "me" and "carcinoma" in the same sentence was like having the arm of God burst through the clouds, yank me up by the throat, and thrust me into the eye of a tornado. I felt immobilized by fear and, at the same time, I experienced an out-of-control whirl of anger.

What kind of physician sends a form letter to notify his patient she has cancer? And the letter was mailed in a nondescript envelope that I almost chunked unopened in the trash can as junk mail.

I sat down on the sofa, letter in hand, and launched into positive self-talk. *Okay, Minda. Breathe in, hold it—one-two-three-four-five-six-seven-eight-nine-ten—exhale. Again. Time for a walk.*

I headed down our mile-long driveway, letter still in hand. I kept rereading it, hoping I had passed over a key word. You do *not* have basal cell carcinoma. No such luck. Each time I read the short letter confirming the diagnosis, my anger deepened. I imagined Dr. P. as an impostor, a lousy excuse for a compassionate healer. He had treated this cancer as nothing more than a harmless wart, ignoring what I had already been through with my tattered medical history. Clip, clip. See you later.

As it turned out, Dr. P. was not far off the mark. The basal cell growth was a minor infraction that hardly deserved the worrisome ranking of cancer. I was at much greater risk of brain damage from falling and hitting my head on a rock than developing an uncontrollable, life-threatening case of basal cell cancer. Yet how was I to know this from his correspondence?

When I got back to the house from my walk, the rolling boil of rage had slowed to a simmer. I called the doctor's office and talked with the nurse. She was calm in response to my now constrained anger. She explained the nature of basal cell cancers—they very rarely cross the confines of the skin.

In an ironic twist of timing, President Reagan was diagnosed with basal cell skin cancer just days *after* I received the ominous letter. However, the front-page news about the cause of his nose boo-boo did not come out until months later, so I missed this lifetime opportunity to bond with President Reagan. It now is almost comical that his spin doctors felt the need to keep the information of his skin cancer under wraps, demonstrating the progress we have made in educating people about the causes and signs of skin cancer.

Five weeks later, a similar growth appeared in the same area adjacent to my other breast. Once again, Dr. P. removed the lesion, and once again, the innocuous-looking tab was basal cell cancer. I was beginning to pay my dues for all that fun in the sun, which with my fair complexion and exposure to the carcinogenic effects of the radiation and CanceRid was more like a scorch under the torch.

1986

The years 1986 to 1988 brought a reprieve from the Cold War tension. During these three problem-free years, I was able to devote my time and energies to mothering, rejuvenating my body with an ample dose of healthy living, and returning to work for the Tennessee WIC Program, known nationally as the Supplemental Food Program for Women, Infants and Children.

This public health nutrition program for low-income mothers and their young children became the birthplace of my professional activism. Assuring that women made an informed choice about saying 'yea' or 'nay' to breastfeeding became a passion I pursued for twenty years—initially within local public health clinics in Tennessee and eventually around the country. The mission to change individual and institutional mindsets began with a pocketful of stamina and a $300,000 federal grant. Through this early work, I was able to document that low-income women could and would choose to breastfeed if given support.

With ample energy and a fire in my belly for life, my activism did not stop with breasts. Bombs unleashed my zeal for justice, too. Nuclear bomb testing to be exact. In 1986, while at an America Public Health Association conference in Las Vegas, I found myself under arrest for protesting underground nuclear bomb testing.

Earlier, I had ridden alongside hundreds of other public health professionals from the conference, on a bus ride to the government testing grounds a couple of hours outside the city. We gathered in the wide-open desert just outside the federal property to await the scheduled bomb test. Carl Sagan, one of the organizers of the protest, enthralled us with a fiery speech until it was time for the countdown. I closed my eyes and listened to Carl's hand-held walky-talky projecting the count into the microphone—10, 9, 8, 7, 6...As I pictured the exploding bomb, the walrus's radiation beams of my teen years came alive once again, and nausea blossomed in my abdomen. 3, 2, 1. The ground rumbled almost imperceptibly under our feet as the blast created a mile-wide crater in the distance.

With this explosion, the US formerly snubbed Soviet President Gorbachev in his appeal for a bilateral one-year moratorium on nuclear testing. I walked arm in arm with my comrades as Carl and his wife led over one hundred of us across the line onto the government property where we were arrested. The charges were ultimately dropped.

Breasts, babies, and bombs – the guiding forces of life during my own peaceful years.

1988

Toward the end of 1988, my body's Cold War resumed with on-again, off-again, swollen lymph nodes in my groin. Once more I found myself on fear watch, as my worry meter rose and fell with the swelling. As a precaution, Dr. Seth Cooper ordered a physical examination every three months.

1989

In 1989, two spontaneous lung collapses diverted our attention from the worrisome nodes. The first incident occurred at home. As I bent over to empty the trash, I felt something shift deep inside my chest, as though a renegade fragment of tissue had broken loose. When I bent again to tie up the garbage bag, the movement recurred. I stood erect, then bent again, testing my body. There it was—a faint, flapping sensation.

An X-ray at Dr. Cooper's office quickly solved the mystery. My lung had sprung a small leak. Dr. Cooper hung the X-ray on the lighted view box, illuminating the fine details of my lungs and ribs. We stood together, staring at the portrait of the inside of my chest.

"There it is," he said, pointing to a barely discernible line on the lower portion of my left lung. "It's a small tear, called a pneumothorax. Looks like about a twenty percent collapse of the lung, meaning you've lost about twenty percent of the function of that lung. Can you see it?"

I had to really focus to see the faint line detected by his expert eyes.

"Yes, right there?" I pointed.

We stared at the X-ray, and Dr. Cooper went out of his way to help me understand. He said, "We have two choices. We can insert a tube into your chest to suck out the air leaking out around the lung. This will allow the lung to re-expand. Or we can just wait and see if it will reabsorb the air and heal on its own."

He waited for a response, but I had none. My mind had wandered into the realm of disbelief, trying to figure out how my body came up with these off-the-wall fractures in health.

He went on to explain the source of this spontaneous collapse. "The radiation you received as a teenager is the most likely cause."

Aha, I thought. *The walrus did it*. Its high-intensity beams scalded my lungs, causing scarring. A scar here, a scar there, had weakened the lung tissue. One too many tugs from the scars eventually created a small tear.

By this time in our relationship, Dr. Cooper was in tune with my desire to err on the side of noninvasive approaches whenever possible. "It's such a small tear, so how about we just wait and see if it will heal on its own?" he said.

I thought the no treatment route was worth a try, and sure enough, in two weeks when I returned to the clinic for another X-ray, the lung was almost fully inflated. Again, we looked at the X-ray together. The line was gone. *That was easy enough*, I thought.

Two months later, it collapsed again. Barry and I were biking in the countryside of Holland outside Amsterdam. Conveniently, it was the next-to-the-last day of a fabulous two-week trip to the low country of Belgium and The Netherlands. No exertion was needed to pedal down the narrow, rural roads of the flat Dutch terrain. Our borrowed one-speed clunkers carried us past gentlemen farmer cottages with fields of sunflowers and gladiolas. I felt great. Then, poof! There she was again—that subtle, but distinctive flapping sensation in my chest.

I stopped my bike. The tires on the well-worn bicycle were in better shape than my lungs. "Yoo-hoo! Hey, Barry!" I tried to get his attention. He was ahead of me several yards up the road.

"What's wrong?" He did a 180-degree turn to answer because, unfortunately, he was much too familiar with my various voices of alarm. He knew something was up.

"I'm ninety-nine percent positive my lung just collapsed again. It's the same feeling I had before."

Experience had taught me that if I bent over to touch my toes, I could actually feel the flip-flopping movement of my deflated lung. "I'm fine," I told Barry.

"It's just a small collapse. I can make it back, but we'd better go now in case it unravels a little farther."

We turned around and very slowly rode the couple of miles back, returning the bikes to the drop-off point at the train station. We wasted no time and headed to the bar for our last Van Vollenhoven Stout to toast a razzle-dazzle end to our Flemish-Dutch excursion. Skol!

Back in Nashville, Dr. Cooper and I stared once again at the newest X-ray.

"There's a line again—in the same place." He pointed to the damage.

"Can we proceed as we did last time and see if it'll heal on its own?" I asked.

"It worked last time. Hopefully it'll work again."

For good measure, Dr. Cooper called Dr. T. at St. Jude to discuss their experiences with radiated survivors. Dr. T. confirmed multiple pneumothoraces were possible. She said they had seen a few patients with this problem, but none had experienced more than two.

A few weeks later, I was back in Dr. Cooper's office, and the fissure was gone. I was getting the impression my body resented its earlier altercations and wanted to remind me who had the upper hand. But when all was said and done, she found a way to move on. In this case, she sealed up the little tear as though it had never happened.

For a while after that, my body's Cold War went into a dormant phase, and my Type-A personality resumed her quest for saving the world, one baby at a time. I began to apply my expertise in public health policy to the national level. Never one to miss an opportunity to question authority, I posed a dilemma to my professional colleagues: *If the US government spends*

*half a billion dollars annually on free infant formula for low
income women, shouldn't it spend a few million helping these
women consider the healthier and cheaper option of
breastfeeding?*

With a small grant from the American Public
Health Association to investigate the issue, I went to
work, and a controversy was launched. After
congressional hearings and help from prominent
politicians, including US Senators Harkin, Leahy and
Dole, the controversy was resolved. Federal funding
and accompanying regulations were approved,
requiring breastfeeding education and support services
for pregnant and new mothers served in public health,
or WIC, programs in all 50 states.

These passionate efforts to seek change in an
expansive way were driven by my cancer experiences.
Instinctively, I had adopted a philosophy to make life
significant while I could. *Do meaningful work. Do it
thoughtfully. Do it well.*

1990

While I was gallivanting around, saving unused
breastmilk, Barry was up to his own mischief back in
Nashville. In addition to a fine job as Shea's father, he
played mandolin and dobro weekly with his rock-and-
roll band Back Creek, and he helped lead the fight to
stop the placement of Nashville's newest landfill in our
pastoral community. We won. The site is now a city
park.

In 1990, Barry and I decided to take advantage of
my good health by setting out on an eleven week
holiday to witness an historic event unfolding
throughout Eastern Europe. In November of 1989, as

political change had begun to rock Eastern Europe, we had watched the news as triumphant East Germans scrambled over the Berlin Wall. We were dumbfounded by this unprecedented event. After more than twenty-eight years, the Communist separation of East and West Germany was coming to an abrupt end. A domino effect occurred with the fall of Communist dominance, breaking down barriers in other Eastern European countries as well.

I felt the urgency to observe firsthand the impact of this grand social experiment. A free market economy grows like a weed, and it would not take long for both the best and baddest of a profit-driven society to obliterate many traces of this period of European history.

At the same time, Barry was transitioning from life as a state bureaucrat to a freelance environmental consultant, while Shea was about to make the big transition from preschool to kindergarten. We were meant to take the summer off.

So in June, 1990, Barry, five-year-old Shea, and I packed our bags. We bookended the eastern leg of the journey with visits to Western Europe to get the full flavor of East and West. Our trip started with a three-week jaunt to Denmark with our friends Inger and Cornelius, and their sons Ian and Dan. We topped off the Danish visit with an excursion to the Danish island of Bornholm. Then in a rented black Ford sedan, we crossed the Baltic Sea on a car ferry into Lubeck in Eastern Germany.

Shea documented the trip with her Polaroid camera, and I felt fabulous as we meandered through the cities and countryside of Denmark and Germany. We reached Berlin just in time for The Wall concert with

Roger Waters of Pink Floyd, The Band, Joni Mitchell,
Van Morrison, Cyndi Lauper, and others. Next we
ventured on to Poland, Czechoslovakia, Austria,
Switzerland, and France.

Shea was a trouper. At age five, she learned to read
maps, frame a scene for a photograph, keep up with
Mom and Dad as we hiked the Tatry Mountains and the
Alps, tour yet another castle, and connect with our
Jewish past via visits to the Nazi death camps where
many of our relatives had perished. Shea became a
seasoned traveler, always ready for the next adventure.
She even played along as her responsible parents hid
wine in her backpack so they could imbibe at The Wall
concert. (It didn't work. They frisked our little
preschooler and confiscated the goods.)

When we returned to the States in September, 1990,
I resumed my job in public health. Barry began his
independent practice as an environmental consultant,
and Shea commenced her formal education at Abintra
Montessori School.

1992

In February of 1992, at the age of thirty-seven, my
Cold War resumed. Seemingly unrelated aches and
pains in my abdomen began to come and go. After
months of watching and waiting for a clear sign of
something serious, Dr. Seth Cooper recommended a CT
scan from my chest to my pelvis to rule out a recurrence
of the Hodgkin's lymphoma. When the scan showed no
evidence of cancer anywhere in sight, we breathed a
sigh of relief. Yet my body was not ready to let me off
the hook.

Jumping out at us from the pelvic scan, like the arrow on a map that says, "You are here," was a tumor on my ovary. Onward to Hospitalization Number Seven and Surgery Number Four, if you are keeping count.

Dr. Cooper was a hematologist whose handiwork focused on disorders of the blood and lymph system. Since this was beyond his expertise, he could only refer me to another doctor. Always careful to suggest physicians with whom I could connect, he said, "Do you have a gynecologist?"

"Yes," I said. "Dr. Barnett helped me deliver Shea, and I like him very much."

Dr. Barnett shared many of the characteristics of Dr. Cooper, traits I found essential for a physician—a gentle, but confident persona, much enthusiasm for the job, and a willingness to participate in a respectful dialogue about various treatments, including possibilities outside the mainstream. When I asked for his honest opinion, I could depend on a frank response without an intimidating edge of superiority.

"Then I suggest you see him right away," Dr. Cooper said. "This is likely just a cyst or benign tumor, but with your history, you shouldn't put this off."

Dr. Barnett's office worked me in right away, which was another good sign of a worthy physician. Even the best and busiest of physicians will work you in once you have an established relationship.

Dr. Barnett gave me an encouraging, but indefinite opinion. "This tumor doesn't look cancerous to me, but we won't know for sure until we get it out. With your history, I think while we're in there we should do a full hysterectomy to remove your uterus, cervix, and both ovaries. Ovarian cancer is sometimes hard to catch early, so it would be a good idea to remove the risk and take out both ovaries."

So much for my vision of a simple tumor removal. With Dr. Barnett's pronouncement that I should say bye-bye to all my reproductive body parts, a litany of questions echoed in my head. The image of butchering healthy body parts when only one chunk was rotten released too many doubts to sort through on the spot.

Am I at risk for uterine cancer? Why remove both uterus and cervix? I don't expect to have more children, but isn't that a pretty hefty chunk of meat to cut out? Are there side effects to leaving a gaping hole? Has research been done on the short- and long-term effects of indiscriminately doing a hysterectomy when the problem is just in the ovary? Would you, Dr. Barnett, remove your testicles if you found a problem only with your prostate?

"Wow, I've got a lot to think about," I told him. "This involves more than I expected." Perplexed and apprehensive, I opted for the easiest way out. Deal with it later.

"How about we schedule the surgery, but let me think about whether I want you to remove just the ovaries or the whole shebang?"

In his graciously soft-spoken way, he replied, "Sure. Just let me know. Call me at any time if you want to talk about it more."

We scheduled the surgery for the following week. In the event it was ovarian cancer, there was no reason to dillydally. So the next day I launched into the research. I visited the Vanderbilt library and called friends in the gynecology business. There was no online Internet surfing yet to both supplement and complicate the research.

I uncovered a few startling findings. First, hysterectomies were routinely recommended by gynecologists when one or more ovaries needed to be removed. Thousands of these elective hysterectomies were performed every year in the United States. Second, I could find only minimal scientific evidence documenting the benefits or possible side effects of this elective surgery. Third and most compelling, one state was considering a law requiring physicians to inform their patients that the additional surgery was elective, supporting my conclusion that insufficient evidence existed to justify the risks.

I made another appointment with Dr. Barnett to discuss my findings. He made no attempt to talk me into the hysterectomy, nor did he make me feel uncomfortable for questioning his recommendations. We discussed my specific risk of uterine cancer. In the years he had been caring for my body, he had observed no fibroid tumors or any other indications that might increase my risk. In regard to the cervix, an annual Pap smear was a very effective, well-documented test for catching cervical cancer early.

I also discussed the dilemma with Dr. Cooper. Unlike Dr. Barnett, he felt my history of cancer was reason enough to proceed with the hysterectomy. A prophylactic surgery would remove one additional possible site for cancer. I told him I appreciated his concern, but I did not agree. He kindly backed off and said he appreciated my perspective as well.

Drs. Cooper and Barnett were two physicians whose opinions I greatly valued. However, their opinions did not trump my research. Rather, the research opened the door to a thoughtful discussion with each of them of the pros and cons *related specifically to my situation.* This deliberation solidified my gut feeling. The fact that neither physician felt the need to pressure me was telling. I'm sure they would have voiced a deeper concern if they were secure in the knowledge supporting their recommendation. So I opted for an oophorectomy, the removal of my ovaries alone.

With the *what* and *when* of the surgery out of the way, it was time to focus on the worst fear, another possible encounter with the cancer demons. Dr. Barnett had laid the groundwork for a positive outlook, and I had a hunch his hunch was right. But I had heard the positive spin before. Ovarian cancer was messy stuff, so I felt an urgency to get to work before D-day.

This time when I sat myself down on my blue zafu meditation pillow, an image formed in a matter of minutes. A Brillo pad scrubbed away on the tumor, and the cast-off cells disintegrated as they fell. Seven days before surgery was not enough time to build a solidly positive frame of mind, yet the visualizing and relaxation lessened my anxiety and helped me stop worrying about that which I could not control.

The hospital stay for Surgery Number Four lasted three short days, and I got off easy. No cancer. Instead, Dr. Barnett found a benign, lemon-sized tumor, but no less conniving than her cancerous distant cousin. In an abysmal feat of immaculate conception, my body had birthed a teratoma, a self-replicating mass of wacky ovarian cells, hair, teeth, bone fragments, and other goop haphazardly tossed together.

The effort to extract the tumor, the tumor's mama (my ovary), and her suspicious sister (my other ovary) was uncomplicated. An annoying hangover, however, was the sudden jump in frequency and intensity of hot flashes. Although my ovaries had never recovered from the CanceRid abuse, they had released enough estrogen to keep my internal thermostat from oscillating totally out of control. But this surgery snipped out the control knob to my thermostat, along with my two motherships of estrogen production. My temperature spiked and plunged, up and down, all day and all night long. My body was screaming for help.

What was a lost girl in the medical Land of Oz to do, but turn once again to one of the Wizards behind the curtain—Wyeth Pharmaceuticals, makers of Premarin.

"Hormone replacement therapy (HRT) is your best option," Dr. Cooper and Dr. K., my new gynecologist, both told me unequivocally. (I had recently switched gynecologists because my new insurance policy no longer covered care with Dr. Barnett.) Both doctors were convinced of the extraordinary benefits this miracle drug offered.

"Supplemental estrogen will get the hot flashes under control. It will decrease your risk of heart disease, *and* it will help prevent osteoporosis," they said.

This same song and dance had been pitched to me for years from every doctor I'd consulted, and now the drumbeat was getting louder and louder. Yet I still believed the manmade, as opposed to womanmade, estrogen-progesterone elixir was just a new version of "Vitameatavegimen," the fictitious cure-all from the "I Love Lucy" show. My two HRT evangelist doctors were taken aback when I replied, "No thanks."

Yet the hot flashes were drowning me in repeated rounds of sweat several times per *hour*. No sooner had my thermostat dropped to normal range and my clothes dried enough to unstick from my skin than my temperature spiked anew, and the entire process repeated itself.

During this vulnerable state, the front-line HRT sales staff, otherwise known as physicians, threatened me with their dire messages of doom if I did not believe. Their gospel had an ominous overtone. "You're too young to go without estrogen. It's been years since your bones and heart have been protected by a normal flow of estrogen."

No other options beyond this drug were ever discussed. Not one. They offered only two alternatives—HRT or a future of broken bones and premature heart attacks. The prevailing wisdom of HRT's virtues was coming at me from all directions, not just doctors. Nurses and friends were convinced of its powers as well. So after years of resistance, I finally did what most women did. I said, "Yes, I'm ready to be saved! Dunk me now! Wash me clean!"

In exchange for the three-inch square of paper from Dr. K.'s prescription pad, I got a pocketful of hormone pills. Within a few days, my hot flashes were gone, and I believed I was saved. I should have known better.

chapter seven

1993

In 1993, a few months after Surgery Number Four, I resigned from a fifteen year tenure with state government and assumed a position as grantwriter, and ultimately, the national coordinator of the US Baby-Friendly Hospital Initiative. This UNICEF/World Health Organization program was being launched around the world in both over- and under-developed countries to improve infant morbidity and mortality rates by overcoming obstacles to breastfeeding in birthing facilities. The head of UNICEF had criticized US health officials for snubbing the program, claiming the Ministries of Health in developing countries were asking, "If US hospitals don't do it, why should we?"

Egged on by several colleagues, I jumped into the fray. We decided to take on the US Department of Health and Human Services, the American Hospital Association, and of course, the multinational infant formula industry. No problem. Following a year of significant progress in advancing our agenda, a thirty-four-page, US government-funded legal opinion declared the UNICEF program a violation of US antitrust laws.

My brave little heart sank. For a day. The next day, this cocky cancer survivor said, *Oh yeah?*

With assistance from friends in the Senate Judiciary Committee, we burned holes in their expensive opinion intended to be the final nay against launching the program in the United States. Two years later, the first US hospital received the official designation as a Baby-Friendly hospital. Over one hundred US hospitals and birthing centers have since met the rigorous requirements for providing the gold standard of care for infant feeding to their maternity patients.

During the first couple of years in this national wrangling over Baby-Friendliness, my body continued to hang in there, allowing me to devote my attention to the world outside the medical maze. The daily dose of hormones seemed like a helpful start each morning. I appreciated the absence of a hot-flash ravaged body, yet my rebellious intellect remained as skeptical as ever.

Popping hormones day after day left me ill at ease. One of my favorite professors in graduate school, Dr. Smith, had warned his disciples to be wary of anything interfering with the delicate handiwork of hormones. As an astute biochemist ahead of his time, he forced us to trail the pathways of the hormones through the body until we understood the elaborate effects of these designer chemicals. We drew lines and arrows to show how one hormone affected another, which affected another, which affected another. The sketches became tangled webs of seemingly random lines that made us cross-eyed. Mother Nature had labored long and hard to create a series of checks and balances to safeguard the entire operating system.

So each day as I swallowed my daily fix, an irksome, indecisive, little voice in my head whispered, *That's probably not a good idea.*

But the sermons from the mounts of my well-educated, well-meaning doctors spoke a lot louder. For more than two years, I dutifully fell in line with their persuasive doctrine—until the line led me directly to another active combat with the cancer demons.

1995, AUGUST

In August, 1995 while on our annual holiday with Barry's family, I lay in our canopied bed in an 1870 bed-and-breakfast overlooking the Berkshires. Barry and Shea had already gone downstairs for breakfast, and I was alone, wallowing in the solitary, stress-free space of vacation heaven. Lying on my back I thought, *I might as well catch up on the monthly self-exam of my breasts.*

I raised my right arm above my head, and with the fingers of my left hand, I applied a gentle pressure on my right breast, performing a clockwise dance around the nipple. My fingers undulated with the steady rhythm of a caterpillar's legs, moving methodically in concentric circles outward from the nipple. My fingertips knew the terrain well. The curious rumba was almost over as I reached the right side of my breast just under my arm. Then my fingers stopped dead still, as though they had a mind of their own.

Holy shit! No! No! I retraced my steps to confirm the discovery. No mistake about it, a pea-sized land mine was buried at the nine o'clock position.

I sat up in the bed as if awakened by a bad dream. I turned toward the night stand, grabbed the bottle of hormone pills, and hurled it into the wicker trash can by the bed. It was a good thing I didn't miss because there was enough anger in my throw to make a permanent dent in the aged pinewood floor.

Anger, shock, and betrayal melded together to send me into a seething trance. My eyes froze, focused on the bare wall beyond the bed. I emerged from the trance a good five minutes later.

"Oooommmmmmm," I chanted. "Breathe in deeply. Hold. Release."

I'm okay, I told myself. *I can deal with this. Trading off the estrogen for a heavy dose of mental imagery is the best place to start. I'll start tomorrow. And I'll see Dr. K. when I get back to Nashville.*

After this pep talk, I pushed the dense cloud of anxiety aside and pulled myself out of bed. As I stood up, I laid both hands on my breast, left hand on top of the right, and gently squeezed—a pleasant, pulsating love offering, taking in the unique vitality of the breast, where softness meets firmness. *My breast, my friend, we're in this together.*

My next thought was, *You're talking to your breast, Minda. Not a good sign.*

I shook my entire body as briskly as a Labrador retriever ridding herself of unwanted bath water. Then I got dressed and headed downstairs to breakfast. I kept the news to myself.

Later in the day, when I passed the hot potato to Barry, he took the news calmly. As an experienced male caregiver who had ridden the ups and downs of my fleshly traumas, he responded in his usual, overly optimistic way. "It will be okay. Don't worry."

(Note to significant others: "Don't worry. It will be okay," is not the response your loved one is reaching for. Would you "not worry" if a lump took refuge in one of your balls? A more helpful reply would be, "Oh, my gosh, not again. What do you think we should do? How can I help?" Acknowledging the fear sets the stage for an honest, productive dialogue about possible next steps.)

In the morning, after opening my eyes and spotting the grave, black cloud blocking my light, I rolled out of bed and sat cross-legged on the floor, buoyed by two pillows to support my spine. I closed my eyes, consciously relaxing my forehead, my eyelids, the corners of my eyes, my cheeks, the corners of my mouth, my lower jaw, my neck, and my shoulders. I inhaled ten slow, deep breaths, followed by a ten-second hold and a slow, deliberate release. I mentally tracked the movement of air as it entered my nose, flowed into my lungs, and expanded my chest and diaphragm. Exhaling, I mentally watched as the air escorted the contaminated gunk out of my body. Random speckles of opaque browns and blacks were expelled with each breath. I could feel and see the movement of each breath and the healing energy it ferried.

With each subsequent in-breath, a warm, soft, golden glow spread throughout my body. Finally, my focus shifted to a deep red-orange layer of icy heat encapsulating the lump. Very slowly I squeezed the lump smaller. It was almost too easy. After about thirty minutes, I could no longer "feel" the heat, so I opened my eyes and stood up.

The next few days, I followed the same routine, rising early enough to start the day with this imagery. I continued the routine when we returned home from vacation. Some days seemed more productive than

others, but over time, the lump seemed to be melting
away like a cube of ice in the sun. *Unlike* a melted cube
of ice, though, there was no puddle left behind, rather a
speck—of what, I'm not sure. A final holdout maybe,
struggling to revive. But the palpable lump was gone. I
was ready for a consultation with Dr. K., the
gynecologist.

"I don't feel anything," Dr. K. mumbled as he
palpated my right breast. He rotated his fingers over
my breast again. "No, I don't feel a mass. How about
sitting up? Let's talk about how to deal with this."

In the typically awkward scene that unfolds after
an intimate examination of private parts with a relative
stranger, I sat up on the edge of the examining table
and closed the gown to cover my breasts. Since he had
not shared anything intimate with me, I felt
subordinated, but I began the dialogue as though
nothing had transpired. After the first couple of
sentences, we were back on equal ground.

Dr. K. posed a suggestion. "I can prescribe a type of
estrogen that may function differently from Premarin. It
will help with the hot flashes but may not effect on the
breast tissue in the same way."

I was so ecstatic that he found nothing suspicious,
and so averse to going back to the wretched days of hot
flashing, I didn't question his recommendation. I
wasted no time reinstating the daily dose of synthetic
estrogen later that day, believing this new version had a
distinctly different mode of action. But a couple of
weeks later, the lump was back.

I immediately stationed myself on the floor for the
daily routine of relaxation and mental imagery, but
unlike the last go-around, the lump seemed rigid and
impenetrable. Day after day, I felt it resisting my effort

like a strong-willed preschooler hunkering down under the kitchen table, refusing to come out and go to bed. Occasionally, I had a faint sense the lump was beginning to succumb. But the next day, her defiance was back. My worry meter climbed higher until I could no longer delay another visit to the doctor. I returned to Dr. K's office.

Lying on the examining table, I lifted my arm behind my head as he massaged my right breast. "I feel it," he said. He palpated my breast again. "Yes, I feel a mass. It's small, but definitely there. Sit up and get dressed, and then let's talk."

He left the room, and I put on my bra and blouse as quickly as I could, anxious to turn the page. When he returned, he strongly encouraged me to have a mammogram as soon as possible, but softened the blow by emphasizing that most of the time these masses turned out to be benign.

The next day, I walked into the waiting room of the Vanderbilt Women's Center, and *all* eyes were glued to the TV set in the corner. A loud hush hung in the air as the zombie-patients sat motionless, staring at the box. The mesmerizing power of the telecast was eerily reminiscent of November 22, 1963. Had President Clinton been shot? Had there been an Oklahoma City copycat bombing?

Yes, someone had been murdered, but it wasn't the president. It did not involve innocent children—directly anyway. The victims were Nicole Brown and Ron Goldman, and this was the final day of the O. J. Simpson trial. The jury would deliver its verdict at any moment, and the TV commentators were commentating about their colleagues' comments ad nauseam.

I joined the spellbound assembly, riveted by the macabre downfall of the rich and famous. I had not been so engrossed by an inane drama since the congressional hearings for Clarence Thomas's Supreme Court appointment.

Minutes passed as we listened to the predictions. At a commercial, I swung back into reality and realized I had not yet signed in. I walked up to the registration window, entered my name on the log, and took a seat.

A few minutes later, the door beside the receptionist's desk opened, and a white-coated young woman mispronounced my name. "Ms. Lazoff?" Apparently, she had never learned phonetics.

I sprung up from the chair. "That's me."

As we walked back to the dressing room, she asked, "Have you ever had a mammogram?"

With my affirmative reply, she spared me the cryptic "how it will feel" description. I took off my shirt and bra and tied on the gown, drifting in the safe zone between optimism and foolish denial. I felt certain this entire event was a false alarm. I'd concocted my Breast Angel Theory, which equaled the absurdity of my Pasteurized Milk Hypothesis from years earlier. According to my theory, breasts were sacred, and because I had already endured so much in the twenty-five years since my original diagnosis, surely my beautiful bosom buddies would be spared. Who or what was doing the sparing I wasn't sure. But in my mind, an Angel of Breasts was keeping watch.

With fears soothed by this conveniently ludicrous theory, I stepped up to the mammogram machine so my nose almost touched its back wall. The technician gently grasped my right breast as if she were coddling a baby bird—a well-fed, size C baby bird—and placed the suspect body part on the metal shelf.

"This may be cold. Here we go. Gonna feel some pressure, but it shouldn't hurt."

She slid the top metal shelf down onto my breast until my flesh lay flattened between the two metal plates like a hamburger in a George Foreman grill. Once again, my guess is men outnumbered women on the design team of the mammogram machine.

"Hold still," she commanded, as if I could make a run for it, leaving my breast behind in the jaws of the lean, mean, grill machine. Then she left the room.

Unable to move, my mind wandered to odd places. Scott, the neighborhood bully from my childhood, leapfrogged ahead of the thousands of more recent memories. He had just tied me to a tree in the Maury woods in the midst of a neighborhood game of hide-and-seek. He left me there all alone shackled to the tree, not a soul within earshot. But Scott was a benevolent bully and returned soon to release me, just as the technician returned to free my breast from the grill.

The tech sent me back to the hallway outside the mammogram room while she, or some other faceless wizard in the bowels of the clinic, perused the images to make sure she got a readable portrait of my breast's internal landscape.

She came back a couple of minutes later with a sheepish look on her face. "We need to do it again. Sorry to make you go through this one more time."

Better to redo this now than to call me tomorrow for a return visit, I reasoned. This second time, the technician moved through the steps with a less robotic handling of the hunk of meat. As she positioned the breast just right, she apologized once again for the repeat performance.

"This should do it," she said. "You can get dressed now and return to the waiting room."

A few minutes later, she called my name again, with the same apologetic look. *Now what?* I thought. *How incompetent can you get?* I was beginning to get a bit rankled. I really didn't want to miss the Simpson verdict.

"Ms. Lazoff, we'll need to do the mammogram one more time. We still don't have it right," she explained.

I did not know then what I know now—having mammograms repeated twice usually means something's up. The real Wizard of Oz, the radiologist, was hiding behind the curtain, reviewing the technician's work to uncover suspicious findings. I was still in the psychic safety zone of the Breast Angel Theory and assumed it was the fault of the technician.

One more time the tech skillfully turned my plump breast into a pancake between the two metal shelves. And once again I got dressed and took my position in the waiting room. The jury had not yet reached a verdict.

The technician reappeared. "Ms. Lazoff? Would you come on back, please?"

Amen, I thought. *I'll get my good news and then return to hear the more important news—guilty or not guilty.*

The technician led me to the Wizard's office. He was waiting for me. I have no recollection of a single feature of the radiologist's face, but his message I remember.

He spilled the beans with little fanfare. "I see a suspicious lesion on the mammogram. It's small, a few millimeters. But you should see your physician right away."

I acknowledged his recommendation, but blew it off and turned the conversation to the O. J. Simpson trial. As we headed together to the clinic room to join in the nationwide trance, the Wizard consoled me, even though, in my numb condition, I didn't need consoling.

"We see quite a few false positives, but you should make sure you see someone right away."

In retrospect, I see that he knew the prognosis and was making a worthy attempt to lighten my load while still encouraging me to follow up. I turned to him and replied rather flippantly, "Oh, I've had my share of false positives. I'm sure this is just another one. But I'll check it out just in case."

The waiting room was heavy with the hush. The group think was palpable—an energy funneled toward the TV screen. The last time I had witnessed a nationwide synchronous "think" was after John Lennon's death on December 14, 1980. Though void of the massive outpouring of grief for our beloved John's death, this event still evoked the same high drama.

The moment arrived. The jury was seated. Judge Ito cautioned everyone to remain calm. As O. J., John Cochran, and the other attorneys rose to their feet and faced the jury, the group trance intensified to a paralyzing hypnosis. Every person in the waiting room sat motionless. Time stood still as Mrs. Robertson, the court clerk, read the verdict.

"In the matter of the people in the state of California versus Orenthal James Simpson, Case Number BA097211, we the jury in the above entitled action find the defendant Orenthal James Simpson not guilty in the crime of murder."

In homes, offices, and Sears appliance centers throughout the United States, the fissures of racial harmony cracked apart. Much to my narrow-minded, whitey surprise, not everyone in the waiting room was aghast. While we white sisters yelled at the box, "What in the hell!" our African-American sisters remained quiet and tense, aware that their relief that a black brother was not, once again, wrongly accused of the death of a white woman might not be well received. Commentators had much to comment about, so they quickly switched the camera from the courtroom to the newsroom. I headed out the door.

When I got home, I called Dr. K., who instructed me to make an appointment for a biopsy with Dr. Jeanne Ballinger, a well-known and highly respected surgeon in Nashville. My attitude was still bolstered by my belief in the Breast Angel, though my theory was not quite impervious to doubt.

I scheduled an appointment for an excisional biopsy with Dr. Ballinger. In this type of biopsy, she would remove most, if not all, of the unwanted tissue. I called my good friend and nurse practitioner Kathleen to accompany me to the outpatient surgery. With her assistance, I would be able to pick up some of the pertinent details I often missed in these visits.

Kathleen and I both knew Dr. Ballinger socially, so we called her Jeanne. We expected a friendly chitchat about the procedure. Instead, after preliminary hellos and updates on our children, Kathleen and I were taken aback by Jeanne's matter-of-fact description of breast cancer treatment options. We exchanged furtive glances in an attempt to determine if the other was equally confused. Although Jeanne said the biopsy might reveal no cancerous cells, the descriptive summary of possibilities in the event of a positive diagnosis was disturbing, particularly given my state of denial.

Mastectomy, lumpectomy, quadrectomy, radiation, chemotherapy. Hey, how about a simple, upbeat response like, *Everything will probably be fine, so go home, relax, and I'll call you tomorrow.*

When Jeanne left the room, Kathleen and I sat together in silence, unable to properly filter the conversation for a result compatible with our original expectations. Jeanne soon returned, followed by a nurse and a rolling metal tray table with the surgical equipment.

The biopsy was just shy of a breeze. Localized injections to numb the area were followed by a one-inch incision which led Jeanne straight to the evildoer. Since the mass was close to the surface, she was able to get in and out in a matter of minutes, causing minimal discomfort.

Kathleen and I walked out of the clinic forty-five minutes after walking in. We were bamboozled. Using my natural talents for persuasive bullshit, I managed to convince myself and Kathleen that we were just caught off guard. Even though Jeanne's talk had been foreboding, we summoned up a rationale: Jeanne was simply being the thorough physician that she is, preparing me for the worst, just in case.

Rationalizing works best in a cloud of ignorance. Neither of us had any idea mammograms could reveal anything firm or definitive. Kathleen and I were forty and forty-two, respectively, too young to have experienced the frequent false and sometimes true alarms of breast cancer experienced by women in their fifties and beyond.

The next afternoon, Jeanne called. "Minda, the biopsy came back positive. I'm so sorry," she said with genuine compassion. How does a physician maintain a sincere inflection during a call like this one made several times a month?

I was silent.

"It's invasive lobular carcinoma, not the most common form of cancer, but not uncommon either."

Translation: Despite what the good folks of Victoria's Secret may believe, breasts exist to make and supply milk. The pathologists found cancerous cells in the lobules of my breast where breast milk is manufactured. They also observed cancerous cells beginning to invade "in a single file fashion" the surrounding tissue of fat and one of the ducts, which are the pipelines for the outflow of milk from the lobules to the nipple.

I was silent.

"Here's the good news," Jeanne said. "I got good margins around the mass, and there were no signs of cancer in the outlying tissue. A very good sign."

Translation: The surgeon removed additional tissue all around the lump to help determine if the cancerous cells had already escaped to more distant territory such as the lymph nodes. This additional information was integral to determining the next steps.

Void of words, I managed a grunt. "Hmmmm."

"Minda, the mass was small, nine millimeters [one-third inch], and it looks like we got it all yesterday. But with your history, we want to make sure. A mastectomy is the next and hopefully final step." She paused, waiting for a reaction.

"I'm listening. Sorry, just trying to digest what you're saying."

"Before we proceed with surgery, I suggest you see an oncologist to discuss the alternatives in the event you need additional treatment. Do you have anyone in mind?"

"No," I replied. One syllable was about all I could muster.

After a pause, I added, "Can you recommend someone?"

"Yes. Dr. C. in Seth Cooper's office."

As I've mentioned, Seth Cooper was my hematologist.

Jeanne continued, "We can talk, too, especially about the surgical options, but this colleague of mine is an oncologist, and he's more familiar with the most updated information regarding the various treatment modalities, especially in regard to your particular situation. You may want to talk with Seth as well."

Silence.

"I realize this is a lot to digest. How about you see Dr. C., and then let's talk? In the meantime, please feel free to call me anytime." As a first-class practitioner dedicated to helping women navigate the medical system, Jeanne always encouraged me to call her.

"Do you have any questions for me now?"

"Thanks, Jeanne, can't think of anything else right now."

I hung up the phone. My hand lingered on the receiver in an unconscious attempt to stop time. The space one resides in after hearing, "You have cancer," resembles a dark closet with no doors, no light, no air. The mind jumps into a defensive mode and goes blank, as if landing in the frame of a cartoon—just having been bonked on the head, with exclamation marks hovering over your head.

Then the door to the closet slowly opens, letting in a crack of light. Behind the light is a flood of questions which, if you are fortunate, quickly get distilled down to, *What should I do next? Who should I turn to?*

Rarely is self-aggrandizing behavior approved in our society, and yet there is no better time to milk friends and relatives for attention than when you have breast cancer. I knew from experience my supporters were the primary source of the strength that would carry me through the ordeal, no matter where it ended. So I wasted no time in hanging out my shingle: SYMPATHY, LOVE, AND ATTENTION WANTED HERE NOW!

Barry was my first victim. He had just returned from work, and I lassoed him before he'd gotten halfway through the kitchen door.

"Jeanne called. The biopsy came back positive. Looks like the breast has got to go."

He was stunned. "Oh, shit. No, Minda. Tell me what she said." He came over and gave me a wooden embrace. His emotions were in the dead zone where mine had been a few hours earlier.

I told him the short story, which was really all I knew.

"Let's not jump to conclusions," he said. "First things first. Let's talk with Seth." (As the years had passed and our familiarity deepened, Dr. Cooper had become Seth.)

"Good idea." A terse response was the limit of my verbal capabilities at the moment.

I dialed the number to make an appointment for a face-to-face consult the next day. When the receptionist answered, I said, "I'm a patient of Dr. Seth Cooper's. I've just been diagnosed with breast cancer and need to see Dr. Cooper as soon as possible."

"Let's see. It doesn't look like I can get you in until next week," she responded, as if I were calling about a stubbed toe. She offered no apologies, no sympathies. She apparently could not hear my need for special attention.

I must be more explicit, I thought. "I'm sorry, you may not have heard me. I was just diagnosed with breast cancer. Next week won't do."

"Let's see here. No, don't think I can get you in any sooner." Not even a faint whiff of an acknowledgment of the Big C diagnosis.

She was not catching my drift. *Now I have the picture*, I thought. *I'm dealing with a communication imbecile who should be placing preformed biscuit dough on a baking sheet at Kentucky Fried Chicken.*

"I'm sorry," I said, no longer able to mask my irritation, which was about to erupt in a torrent of unfeminine language. "You're not listening. I have breast cancer. Breast cancer, got it? I just got the news a few minutes ago. I've been a patient of Dr. Cooper's for sixteen years, and I need to see him *right away.*"

"I'll have to call you back," she replied. Still no hint of apology. Instead, she sounded frustrated that I was violating her Roberta's Rules of Appointment Order.

I fought back the tears with only my anger checking a very upsetting sense of hopelessness.

"Forget it!" I shouted. And I hung up.

Barry was standing by and overheard the increasing decibel and frustration level on my end of the conversation. Before I even finished the call, he already had our compassionate friend Joe Ingle on the other phone line. Joe was the husband of Seth's nurse practitioner, Becca, and within five minutes, he called back to say that he'd arranged an appointment with Dr. C. for the next day, and that Seth himself would call us momentarily.

Our conversation with Seth was brief but comforting. The sound of my medical partner's voice moderated my rising wave of jitters. Seth said he would call Jeanne and get right back to me. And he did. He confirmed the lump was small and caught early. He hoped for and expected the best.

He said, "You'll be in excellent hands with Dr. C. He and Jeanne work closely together. And you probably already know Jeanne's the best."

I felt like malleable putty, ready to fit myself into any chink of hope. Emotional fatigue had conquered my usual skepticism and erased my ability to question authority. I chose the easy road. Just do it.

"Thanks, Seth. This is just what I needed to hear. I feel better."

Once again, I felt grateful for the emotional healing power of a physician who held my trust and confidence. Having a medical advisor as my confidant in time of need—someone who returned my call right way and who saw the whole picture, even if we didn't always agree—was a critical pillar of support.

Though I had calmed down, at least superficially, Barry was fully aware of my fragile state. He did something he rarely did. He cancelled his appearance with his band for that evening. By the next morning when Barry and I showed up for the consultation with Dr. C., we were wearing our steel armor, faking readiness to hear the worst. The doctor explained that, with my history of cancer and radiation, a mastectomy was my best and possibly only option.

"I wish I could give you more options," he said. "Less radical surgery requires follow-up radiation, but Seth and I talked this morning, and we agree you're not a candidate for more radiation. You've already received a lot of radiation as a teenager, which may have contributed to this cancer."

Barry and I humbly offered no response.

He continued, "In order to determine if the cancer has moved beyond the breast, Jeanne will also remove some fat around your armpit along with the lymph nodes draining your breast."

Dr. C. lightened the impact of this news by expounding on his guess of the prognosis. "The margins around the mass were clean of cancer, so if our assumptions are correct and the cancer was caught early, we will find no cancer in the lymph nodes. No cancer in the nodes means no chemotherapy."

I was elated to hear that whacking off my fat-laden mammary glands could replace the need for the prolonged chemo torture. I had been shivering in my sandals at the thought of mainstreaming more noxious chemicals. *Surgery only—no chemo—I can handle this*, I thought.

Barry, however, had a drastically different reaction. Life without one of his wife's breasts was a burden he was not ready to bear. As we left the clinic and walked toward the car, he spoke emphatically, "There has got to be another way."

While Barry was cogitating over this, a few of Dr. C.'s words echoed in my head: *The radiation you received as a teenager may have contributed to this cancer.*

Did I hear right? Had my youthful Pasteurized Milk Theory gone sour? Had the Breast Angels never protected me at all? A feeling of betrayal began to slither up my spine. *I must talk with Seth*, I thought.

Barry was steering his angst in another direction. When we got home, he immediately kicked off his campaign to rescue my breast from the chopping block. His reaction provided timely comic relief. He had not flinched when my ovaries were slated for the can. Nor had he taken an active role in researching the treatment for my relapse of Hodgkin's disease. Neither shingles nor infertility drew this reaction. In the past, my own medical choices had reigned supreme, with no need for intervention on his part beyond emotional support. The difference between then and now was a breast.

In his defense, he was not only concerned for the obvious reasons. He was also rightly questioning why an entire appendage had to be amputated when most, if not all, of the cancer had already been removed. So he donned a cape and flew into action.

After a series of calls, he was directed to a breast cancer center at the University of Pittsburgh Cancer Institute. A real live nurse answered his call. Her sole job was to answer questions about breast cancer. He conversed with her for more than an hour about my diagnosis, the various treatments, and the current recommendation for a mastectomy. Once she heard about my history, she concurred that mastectomy was probably the only choice.

Despite the stark and stinging contrast between Barry's earlier lack of motivation and his newly found eagerness to dive into the trenches of the research, I was thankful for all the help I could get. Maneuvering my way through the medical maze demanded time, stamina, and persistence to ask the right questions of the right experts, and it was refreshing to see Barry actively gathering data.

Much to his disappointment, Barry's Save the Breast campaign reached a dead end. While he was consulting with the breast lady in Pittsburgh and other experts in Nashville, I contacted Seth again. Both routes led to the same conclusion. To save Minda, get rid of the breast. And for good measure, we may want to consider getting rid of the other one, too.

For the moment, I was oddly at ease with the impending loss of one or more breasts. I could handle surgery, but enduring more rounds of CanceRid was the repulsive option I wanted to avoid at all costs. Loss of a breast to minimize the need for months of vomiting, diarrhea, and extreme fatigue—this was an easy choice. I remained perplexed, however, by the irony that my cancer radiation treatment twenty-five long years ago had left my bosom buddies ripe for more cancer demons.

Seth wisely steered me toward reconciliation with the staff at St. Jude Children's Research Hospital. Who better to consult about this dilemma, he counseled, than my estranged medical confidants who now had two more decades of research under their belts?

After the St. Jude staff had left my Hodgkin's recurrence unchecked for almost a year, I had seen little value in seeking out their expertise again, and over the past few years, our communications had extended no further than the questionnaire mailed to me every fall. Their survey asked about my state of health—any new cancers, surgeries, problems, or procedures over the previous year. I usually let the survey sit a while, ambivalent about maintaining a tie to the past. Inevitably, though, I completed and returned each survey.

In retrospect, the regularity of this data-gathering provided me with a sense of assurance. The surveys from St. Jude, my long lost guardian, in conjunction with the annual exams with Seth and my zeal for healthy living, led me to believe I was in touch with the most current information regarding my risks and modes of prevention for possible problems.

While I was floating on this dubious cloud of self-confidence, the data were streaming in from around the country about the latent effects of childhood cancer treatment. The results showed women my age who had stacked up twenty-plus years of living after the original radiation and chemical onslaught were particularly at risk.

When I called St. Jude, the first personal contact with the staff in fifteen years, I was connected to Dr. Melissa Hudson. Dr. Hudson was the director of the After Completion of Therapy Program, or ACT Clinic. Had I been more observant, I might have noticed the name of this newly established clinic on the cover letter of the annual surveys. Instead, I had unwisely maintained my distance from an international repository of knowledge on childhood cancers. Like a rebellious adolescent, I held onto my independence from those authorities.

The breast cancer was no surprise to Dr. Hudson. "We're seeing more and more cases of breast cancer among Hodgkin's survivors, particularly patients like you who received radiation to the chest as a teenager."

Again, I was stupefied. *Why hadn't anyone told me?*

Having met Dr. Hudson only over the phone, I withheld my emotionally laden questions and focused on the new information. As Dr. Hudson and I discussed the recent data substantiating the increased risks of breast cancer among long-term Hodgkin's survivors, her enthusiasm for the subject and her sincere interest in my well-being resonated throughout our conversation. Dr. Hudson was a fast talker, so she covered a lot of ground in a brief span of time.

"Why don't you send the slides to me, and I'll have one of our pathologists look at them?" she said. "We would like to see the slides anyway for our records."

"Wonderful! A second opinion would be most helpful," I replied. "I've been told they think they got it all, yet they recommend a mastectomy. My husband is very upset and doesn't understand why I can't have less radical surgery. The lump was so small. Do you think a mastectomy is necessary?"

"Unfortunately, in your situation, I agree with them. There is probably no alternative. We're still learning about the long-term risks, but from what we know now from Hodgkin's survivors, not just here at St. Jude, but from all over the country, the risk for a recurrence in that breast will be too high. The safest approach is to remove the entire breast."

Her opinion was delivered with certitude. In time, I came to learn that Melissa was so intelligent, knowledgeable, and passionate about her work that her switch was always set on high. Her responses teetered on a manic edge—in a good way, a very good way that instilled confidence when I most needed it.

For an instant, my thoughts darted to the "good" breast, but I chose not to go there. *One breast at a time*, I thought. "Thank you so much for talking with me. I feel silly that I've been out of touch all these years. I'm so glad I found you."

Dr. Hudson wasn't through yet. She went on to encourage my participation in St. Jude's follow-up program for survivors. She explained the ACT Clinic was established to help keep tabs on the long-term effects and to get this new information to St. Jude alumni and our health care providers. The data collected from survivors like me were contributing a vast amount of knowledge to the international pool of information on the long-term effects of treatment for childhood cancer survivors.

She said, "The ACT staff is available to help at any time."

I felt like a runaway reconnecting with my long lost guardian who held dark secrets about my insidious lineage. This stranger was devoted to my well-being, with no grudges or constraints. I was reluctant to sign off and sever the tie to this fountain of knowledge, but I bid her good-bye, assuring her I would be in touch.

I hung up, feeling foolish. What other vital information had I missed by harboring resentment toward a noble institution that was still working every day to extend my life? I shuddered as I heard the cracking of my long-held illusion of control.

The conversation with Dr. Hudson helped me grasp the urgency of the current mission: to get rid of the breast. My breast's exterior facade still held a vibrant beauty, but her interior sheltered a smoldering fire poised to ignite the entire neighborhood. The house must be destroyed. But should the next-door unit be destroyed as well?

Another visit with Dr. Jeanne Ballinger ended the debate. Sitting face-to-face in her clinic room the next day, I asked Jeanne directly, "What would you do if you were in my situation? Would you remove both breasts?"

I think she answered more as a friend than my doctor. "It's such a personal decision. In my situation, I would have a double mastectomy. But my mother and paternal grandmother had breast cancer, so my situation is different. Some women feel they would be worrying all the time about cancer in the other breast, while others feel it's too drastic to remove the other breast when there is no evidence of cancer. It's very much a personal choice."

If you are lucky and the planets align just so, there comes a point in the decision-making process when the mode of action is clear. Rarely does this happen unless you place total, naïve faith in your doctor's recommendation. This time around for me, however, I felt there was no room for misinterpretation. The correct answer was, remove Breast Number One, and give amnesty to Breast Number Two.

My rationale for Breast Number One? If a few cells unequivocally demonstrated a propensity for mutating, could the neighboring cells, exposed to the same insidious radiation, be far behind? Time was on their side, not mine.

Rationale for Breast Number Two? None. Just keep the damn thing for my partner's and my own sexual well-being, and hope for the best.

Though my mind was made up, my husband, Mr. Thou-Shalt-Covet-Thy-Wife's-Breasts, was still pleading for the lives of Breasts Number One *and* Two. Barry was indeed disappointed by my decision, but he accepted the edict. Together we were ready to move on to the next decision—to reconstruct or not to reconstruct.

chapter eight

1995, NOVEMBER

As we sought more details about breast reconstruction, doctors and friends directed us to Dr. S., a plastic surgeon at Vanderbilt Medical Center. The nurse escorted us to the examining room and presented us with a scrapbook of the Best of the Best, a parade of topless, aging women proudly posing for the camera to show off their new wares. The nurse encouraged us to peruse both the before and after photographs while waiting for the sculptor.

As Barry and I flipped through the pages of these bare-chested ladies, we were struck by how unlovely most of the models were. With high expectations about the advanced techniques of plastic surgery, both of us imagined forty-something cancer victims with twenty-year-old breasts. The photographs told a different story. Many of these women, beyond the first half century of their lives, had one breast replaced with a facsimile and the twin sister surgically tugged at here and there to match the impostor. The final product was not too bad in most cases, but still lacking beauty.

"Not too bad" is the common response when you tell folks you are recovering from a bad car accident. "Why, you don't look too bad." Translation: You look a little rough, but you could look a heck of a lot worse.

Dr. S. arrived, introduced himself, and launched into a graphic description of the various ways he could reconstruct my breast. I'll spare you, the reader, his euphemistical medical jargon. In layman's terms, this most popular method of creating a mound-like protrusion on your chest was to insert a bag under the chest muscle. The bag's soft, rubbery silicone shell would be filled with either harmless salt water or, according to some, potentially dangerous silicone gel.

Dr. S. did not discourage silicone gel. He was truly sold on the realistic look and feel of silicone. The salt water version made for a forever perky mound, but was not as squeezable and lifelike as its riskier cousin. Nevertheless, although the heat of the silicone implant controversy had passed, the risks of silicone gel were still suspect to me.

The second more complicated method he described was called a TRAM (transverse *rectus abdominis* muscle) flap. Skin and fat from the lower abdomen would be carefully cut and moved up the chest through a tunnel, while blood flow from neighboring vessels would keep the tissue alive. This method required a four- to six-month healing period, but the mound would be made of living tissue from your own body. It would grow and shrink with your changing weight and would feel more natural than an implant. The disadvantage—you would hurt like shit for several weeks, maybe months, as the stretched and severed abdominal muscles screamed in pain the moment you attempted to get out of bed. Further, on rare occasions, infection could get out of control or the tissue might reject its new home and die, in which case the tissue would be removed and the patient could try again or pursue a different method.

A third alternative was based on variations of the other methods, such as an implant plus a back muscle, or fat and a back muscle with no implant. The fourth option—no reconstruction at all—was never mentioned. Every doctor, including the oncologist, assumed I would have mounds installed.

In my mind, it boiled down to three choices— Bag Lady with faux implants, Bionic Woman with my own transmogrified living tissue, or Amazon Mama. Amazon women were a tribe of female warriors in Greek mythology who cut or burned off one of their breasts in order to master the bow and arrow. Their name derived from *a-mazos*, meaning without a breast.

With four notches on my belt for major surgeries, I was not anxious to test my courage again. The Bionic Woman was *definitely* outside my tolerance level. Bag Lady perhaps was worth consideration, although my overly analytical mind asked, *Is it wise to insert a bag in your chest?* I conjured up images of wounded, raw tissue left behind when the breast was removed, and my helpless chest cried out for mercy: *Give me time to heal. You can always stick the bag in later.*

Tinkering with my healthy bosom buddy to match the impostor was troubling as well, yet without an adjustment, the unmatched set seemed to defeat the purpose. The final decision was easy. Keep it simple. One step at a time. Remove the breast. Then let time heal the wounds. If Amazon Mama doesn't work out, we could beckon the Bag Lady.

Drs. Ballinger and Cooper supported my decision.

A few days before the surgery, I told Marshall, a good friend and anesthesiologist, about my decision, and he shared his views to help quell my anxiety. As a participant in surgeries on a daily basis, he had been very impressed with the relative ease of a mastectomy. Separation of the mammary tissue and fat from the surrounding tissue was not a complicated procedure, he said.

I appreciated Marshall's intent to dilute my worry, but I remained skeptical. Easy for the surgeon did not necessarily mean easy for the patient. Having weathered the aftermath and immobilization of abdominal surgeries before, I could not relate.

The night before the surgery, dear friends Ava and Kathleen joined our little nuclear family of three by the fireplace. We held hands as they channeled their healing energy to my breast and heart, and I felt loved and lucky to have such devoted friends and family.

On Thursday, November 16, 1995, I entered St. Thomas for a modified radical mastectomy of my right breast. All parts of the right half of my milk production system—the lobules, ducts, nipple, and areola—and the supporting fat and lymph nodes, connective tissue, and blood vessels were to be removed by Dr. Ballinger. The muscles and outer skin would be left intact.

In the days prior to Surgery Number Five, I'd been so wrapped up in the enormity of the decision-making that I had not cleared out head space to ponder the philosophical questions regarding my self-worth sans my bosom buddy. So as I lay on the gurney in the pre-op room, I muttered my good-byes to Breast Number One as if to a loved one. Why is it that when we lose them, they suddenly feel like beloved best friends?

For twenty-five years, she had been my close companion, luring the opposite sex and elevating my self-confidence. She'd made me feel attractive and deserving of attention. Sorrow crept in as I finally acknowledged the loss I was about to experience, and I felt soaked in self-pity.

While I awaited my turn to be strolled into the operating room, I looked around to see if there were any comrades stewing in a parallel misery. Lying in the gurney on my left was a man a few years older, perhaps fiftyish. I glanced at him to check for any sign of interest in sharing a pre-op moment of reflection. Was he losing a private part? I kind of hoped he was so I would have some company in my eleventh-hour grieving. But his vacuous stare said, "No disturbance wanted."

A white board on the wall behind the bustling nurses' station summarized the surgical stories about to unfold: bed number in the holding area—patient name—doctor—type of procedure. There were several other surgeries on the docket—hernias, gallbladder removals, and appendectomies. I was the only mastectomy. There was no clue about who the guy next to me was, but no penile or prostate victims were listed.

I was bemoaning my solitude in this emotional wasteland when Kathleen appeared to bestow an affectionate bon voyage. "Hi," she said, leaning over the gurney's guardrail to give me a kiss on my forehead.

Like lovers exchanging final good-byes, we locked gazes, and I punctuated the parting with a tender insight. "This sucks!"

The anesthesiologist interrupted our delicate communion. The last thing I remember before the la-la juice took effect was seeing Kathleen's saddened eyes and strained smile.

As it turned out, Marshall's assurance of the relative simplicity of the surgery was right on target. Just hours afterward, I sat up in the hospital bed to welcome friends and family who marched through my room to shower me with flowers, love, and condolences. My postsurgical days were uneventful, and the soreness was easily managed with mild narcotics.

Our society places immeasurable value on youthful sexuality, which for women is epitomized in the breasts. Juxtapose this with the dignity and courage required to face *The Cancer*, and you are transformed into a hero. Few opportunities in life bring forth such focused attention and adulation as recovery from breast removal—regardless of the cancer's size or show of force.

In actuality, I felt like a fraud. My cancer had been contained, and the surgery was comparatively mild. I would be spared the debilitating treatment of chemo, the embarrassing affront of baldness, and the fear of pain and death. Yet to my friends and family, I was their stalwart soldier. This put me in an awkward position of choosing between two personas—the flippant patient in denial of my loss, or the gracious brave survivor. True, the cancer could have been life-threatening, but since it was detected in its very early stages, I was not expecting bad news. So as the well-wishers strolled in and out, I proudly wore my *Big C* arm band and lapped up the attention.

The day after the mastectomy, I learned there was no evidence of cancer in any of the nodes or breast tissue, and the mastectomy made a chance of a recurrence highly unlikely. Now the only justifiable misfortune to grab some pity from friends and family was the immobility of my right arm anchored by two flexible plastic drains siphoning off the excess fluid. Even though the butchering of my breast, most of which was fat, was probably easier than cutting up a roasting hen, a few representatives of the rest of my living body reacted to the slaughter. My immune system was deploying too much lymph fluid and white blood cells in an attempt to heal the wound. So the tubes were inserted to drain the excess and speed up the healing.

On day three prior to discharge, I was shocked back to reality when the bandage was removed. As the nurse gently pulled the gauze away from my sensitive skin, my pulse quickened. Where my breast had been, I saw an orderly row of white Steri-Strip surgical tapes crossing over the incision. There was no bloody jagged gash or gaping hole, just a flat spot with a line across the middle. For once, horrific expectations worked to my advantage. I had anticipated a hideous mutilated chest, so this sight actually brought me relief.

Before I was sent home to fend for myself, the nurse gave me instructions for mobilizing the arm, cleansing the drains, and changing the bandage. I left the hospital in a physically altered state, whittled into a one-breasted Amazon Mama with hollow reeds implanted to leach my body of onerous humors.

As soon as I got home, I slid into my own bed in my forested retreat to be coddled by my tribal sisters and brothers. Ava, Reva, Kathleen, Debbie, Bob, Becca,

Joe, Danny, Brenda, Ann, Rebecca, Sharon, and Alan cooked and cleaned while I read, ate, slept, and healed. Once a day, the nursemaid-in-waiting stripped my reeds of any blockage draining from the underarm wound and emptied the bag of waste.

The tugging and pulling during surgery to separate surrounding tissue had shocked my muscles and tendons, so I was unable to raise the traumatized arm more than a few inches. My arm was as obstinate as a dog on a short rope leaping to chase a rabbit, then abruptly halted in midair by the rope. After a few days at home, I attempted to stretch the rope a tiny bit. I stood in the shower facing one corner with feet planted, arms bent and hands placed against the walls. Very slowly, I moved my chest toward the corner. Then I moved my hands up a couple of inches and repeated the movement. (Later, I learned I was not supposed to begin the stretching until *after* the tubes were removed.)

By midweek, I was walking around the yard, gradually reentering the world. Other than an immobilized arm and a bout of constipation from the anesthesia and pain medication, I felt pretty good. Pretty good for a newly initiated Amazon Mama. Toward the end of week two, I returned to Jeanne's clinic for the post-op visit.

"Looks like you're healing well," she said. "How much fluid have you drained off in the last couple of days?"

"It has really tapered off. Yesterday I drained about twenty cc's."

"Good. If we take the tubes out, you'll be able to do additional exercises to help get your arm moving."

Like most postsurgical patients, I was toddling my way back to health and normalcy, craving praise for each small step, and Jeanne offered the approval she knew I needed. Still, I felt apprehensive about removing the tubes. How was Jeanne going to get those tubes out of my arm? They had begun to feel like extensions of my body, melding themselves to whatever lay beneath my skin. When I moved, the tubes moved.

"Is this going to hurt?"

"It may be a quick ouch, but it shouldn't be too bad."

"All right. Let's get it over with."

"This will just take a second," she said. "Can you move your arm to the side a little? That's it. Here we go. One, two, three."

She dislodged the first tube before I even had a chance to tense up. It felt exactly like you think it would feel, like a foreign object loosely attached with an adhesive bandage had been ripped away from the tissue inside my underarm. The thought of the rip was much worse than the rip itself.

I was just starting to ponder the lack of the pain when Jeanne asked, "Ready for the next one? Move your arm. Ready. One, two three," and she pulled out the next tube.

In the time it takes to yank away two big Band-Aids, we were done. It was well worth the brief discomfort to have a mobile arm again. The excess baggage had been more cumbersome than I had realized. My arm squealed for joy as it was freed from bondage.

"You're looking good. The next step is for you to see Dr. C. again to talk about where we go from here. There's a new drug that could help minimize your risk of a recurrence in your other breast. It's called tamoxifen. Dr. C. will tell you more about it."

We hugged, and I was on my way. What a great lady.

Two days later I met with Dr. C. again. With his gentle, nonthreatening bedside manner, he wasted no time giving me the good news, followed by the not so good news.

"The risk of recurrence in the chest where the breast was removed is negligible, practically nonexistent. Your risk of cancer in the other breast is the concern at this point."

No cancer in the lymph nodes, no need for mainstreaming chemo toxins directly into my veins. Hallelujah! Stopping these demons early on in their assault dramatically reduces the length and intensity of the battle. Still, since the chest radiation I'd had years earlier magnified the risk in my remaining breast, Dr. C. recommended offensive strategies to help keep the insidious demons in check. And in the proactive warfare waged by the modern medical system, the hero would be another pharmaceutical god, Zeneca, the creator of tamoxifen.

"Tamoxifen," Dr. E. said, "is an oral medication especially effective in decreasing the risk of a recurrence in patients like yourself who are estrogen-receptor positive."

I had never heard the phrase "estrogen-receptor positive." The only two people I knew who'd had breast cancer were Chickie and Saralee, my mother-in-law and my sister's mother-in-law, both of whom were treated many years earlier, before this test was available.

He elaborated, "It has to do with the sensitivity of your tissue to estrogen. A positive response for this test indicates you're a good candidate for tamoxifen. This drug minimizes the risk of a recurrence by blocking the estrogen receptor sites of your breast cells."

In laywoman's terms, since I tested positive for estrogen receptivity, we now knew estrogen could function like a key in a lock, opening the doors for havoc in the cells of my lobules and ducts. Once the doors were open, my breast cells could start an orgy of cancerous reproduction, but tamoxifen would lock the doors so estrogen no longer had access.

Dr. C. tossed out one caveat. "You can take it only five years because recent studies have found long-term use beyond five years increases the risk of uterine cancer. It also had been found to increase the incidence of blood clots."

I explained my aversion to taking any more medications than absolutely necessary and that I wanted to think about it.

"No problem. Let's talk again whenever you're ready."

Within a few weeks, four physicians delivered to me the same sermon about the potentially life-saving value of tamoxifen, with the same encouragement about the convincing data, and the same caveat about the five-year term limit. It was the wonder-drug-of-choice for breast cancer patients with estrogen positive receptors, given at the end of treatment for good measure.

To my cynically scarred mind, the unanimous pitch was a red flag. *Caveat emptor.* In the practice of medicine, a phenomenon occurs wherein a critical mass of conviction emerges for a well-marketed medication. Openness to critical reviews of the literature and the possible unknowns become buried under this inflated mass concurrence. Evangelists for the drug often become blind proponents, no longer looking at patients as individuals or actively curious about possible reactions and side effects. When well-intentioned healers hear the same drumbeat of medication wonders day in and day out from people whose judgment they trust, they begin to repeat the message to their patients. After they've invested a huge chunk of their credibility, it becomes hard to stand back and question the validity of that judgment. Consequently, a drug which may have legitimate benefits for *many* people is transformed into a panacea for *all*.

For some patients, this consensus instills confidence. My skepticism takes me in the opposite direction. Like the morning glory that intuitively closes up when the afternoon sun reaches a precise intensity, my mind automatically switches into Question Authority Mode when I hear too many eerily similar messages from different sources. Further, my willingness to believe becomes even more suspended when a drug skyrockets to celebrity in only a few short years.

After hearing the tamoxifen sales pitch from several docs, I elevated a healthy dose of cynicism into two overriding sets of questions. First, since I could take the drug only five years, would I be back to square one when I stopped, or did the miracle worker continue its job forever, even after I stopped taking it?

Second, since this drug was relatively young in its widespread use, did we really know the long-term effects? Many years are needed to understand long-term effects, especially with a chemical interfering with the action of a hormone likely to have impact on other parts of the body. The possibilities for mischief were limitless. The rigorous study required by the US Food and Drug Administration *before* the drug could hit the market obviously helped identify a few risks, but certainly not all.

Clinical trials had shown that tamoxifen *increased* the risk of uterine cancer after five years of use, hence the instruction to limit the term of use. Five years times millions of potential customers might help temper the stockholders' fears, but not mine. How about that magical number? If you stop at five years, are you safe? What about the risk at four years? Three years?

My final verdict: the potential short-term benefit was not worth the potential unknown risks. I told Dr. C., "Thanks, but no thanks for now."

With that decision, my relationship with Dr. C. was over.

So far, I had escaped this confrontation with the cancer demons with just one relatively simple major surgery and the loss of one body part. I was ready to move on to the next dangling worry. What other ominous effects loomed ahead thanks to the radiation the walrus had zapped at me a quarter of a century earlier? Radiation had helped save my life, but were its cumulative effects now stealing my life? The rest of the story lay waiting to be revealed in Memphis. A trip to St. Jude, my former home away from home, was long overdue.

Barry and I hit the road to Memphis during the winter holidays to visit St. Jude and uncover the latest scoop on this double agent called radiation. After dropping Shea off at Barry's parents' home, we drove downtown, and my first glimpse of St. Jude in fifteen years was disorienting. The campus had grown from a few unassuming, low buildings to a sprawling campus of towers, parking lots, and guard stations. We drove back and forth down Danny Thomas Boulevard searching for the hospital's main entrance. Who were all of these people inside these buildings, and what were they doing?

When we finally found the new entrance, Barry dropped me off and left to park the car. As I spun through the revolving door, old memories switched on a high voltage of fear. I took a few steps into the hospital lobby, then stopped. I had just crossed into a house of horrors *and* a safe haven. Here lay the single greatest source of knowledge about my past, present, and future, and I suddenly felt a clash of emotions. The tears rolled down as I pondered the significance of this institution which had altered my existence these past twenty-five years.

Whoa, Nellie, I thought, *what am I about to get myself into?* If I could have turned myself inside out, I would have looked like a mass of wires, crossing and wriggling every which way, desperately seeking order.

By the time Barry arrived, I had begun to adjust to the shock, the bright lights, and the unleashed bundle of memories. I said, "This is weird. Really weird. I'll tell you about it later. Let's go find Dr. Hudson."

We approached the reception desk. "I'm here to see Dr. Melissa Hudson."

"She's in the After Completion of Therapy Clinic."

"The what?" I asked. Her words had rolled right past me, sounding as garbled as the drive-through voice box at Burger King.

"The After Completion of Therapy Clinic," she repeated. "Turn left up ahead. After passing through another waiting area for the leukemia and transplant clinics, turn left again to the receptionist's desk for the specialty clinic."

We thanked her and headed out. Walking down the hall felt friendly, familiar. Even though the building had been remodeled from a drab institutional edifice into a stately clinic with modern furniture and colorful wall paintings of a jungle, the authentically warm and fuzzy St. Jude ambience still pervaded the halls.

Only one preteen and his parents were waiting in the lobby of the specialty clinic. It was December 21, and the clinic was open for limited appointments only. I had called Dr. Hudson from Nashville, and she offered to see us as soon as we got to town.

I checked in at the receptionist's desk. "I'm here to see Dr. Hudson."

Unlike other clinics I'd known, we were escorted straight to an examination room. No one asked for my insurance card. There were no papers to sign guaranteeing payment. Nor were we held in another waiting room to flip through dated *Highlights* magazines while an additional thirty minutes went by. Almost at once, Melissa Hudson flew into our exam room with an animated welcome.

After a brief exchange of pleasantries, she spent the next hour examining me and taking a detailed medical history of the last seventeen years—since my last bout with Hodgkin's lymphoma. She also explained the mission of the ACT Clinic.

"When you first moved away, we had no structure in place to regularly communicate with our patients who had completed treatment, so we lost touch with a lot of patients like you."

I nodded, listening.

"On occasion," she continued, "especially after we started the annual surveys, we would hear back from one of our survivors. They were usually calling for the same reason you called me. They had developed another cancer, an infection, or other serious health problem, and wondered if there was any connection to their initial cancer."

She paused to catch a breath, then kept going.

"Through these calls and the alumni surveys," she said, "we began to see some trends in health problems. Meanwhile, as childhood cancer survivors from the sixties, seventies, and eighties were getting older, other childhood cancer centers around the country were observing similar trends."

"What kind of trends?" I asked.

"Some of these problems were disturbing," she admitted, "particularly second cancers and cardiovascular problems. We decided to pool our efforts and establish an international consortium of research centers to get a better handle on the long-term effects. There are now countless longitudinal studies under way on the latent effects of childhood cancer treatment."

Barry and I listened in awe of her energy, knowledge, and enthusiasm. She was the medical version of Al Gore, hot on the trail for solutions to an unfolding calamity.

"In 1984, St. Jude started the ACT Clinic to keep in touch with our alumni, answer your questions, and gather accurate information about problems experienced following the treatment. Our goal is to educate our alumni about the risks *as* we learn about them. The sooner we can get the information to you and your doctors, the more likely you are to catch these problems in their early stages."

Then, in a gentle move from the general to the specific, Melissa began to share what they knew about female Hodgkin's survivors—increased risks of thyroid cancer, heart attacks, infertility, sepsis . . .

"We now have a cohort of female Hodgkin's patients who have survived fifteen, twenty, even twenty-five years. We're seeing more and more breast cancer among survivors like you who received radiation as a teenager. In fact, evidence shows thirty-five percent of female Hodgkin's survivors who live twenty to twenty-five years after the radiation are developing breast cancer. And the longer this cohort lives, the higher this percentage will go."

She took another quick breath, then said, "It's reasonable to expect you may get breast cancer in the other breast."

I sat back in my chair, not quite ready to absorb her words.

"Today, we don't use nearly as much radiation or chemotherapy as we did when you were treated. Also, we use a different kind of radiation, and we know a lot more about shielding the breasts. I know this doesn't help you feel any better now that you've had breast cancer, but we've learned a lot from you and other patients treated in years past."

I shifted in my seat. "I'm definitely a bit shocked that I wasn't aware of this risk. At least it's good to know what I'm up against." Then I added, "It's wonderful to hear there's a concerted effort to identify the risks for people like me."

The news of the risk to my other breast fell on deaf ears for those few minutes as I quickly acknowledged there was nothing I could do about it now that the surgery was behind me, so I moved on to another issue. "As you were talking, I realized this is a great opportunity to share survivors' challenges not just with their physical health, but with their emotional health as well. Have any survivors talked about their fears of a recurrence? The reason I'm asking is, when I walked into this place, I was reminded that my greatest fear is having to go through chemo again."

Melissa nodded, encouraging me to go on.

"For me," I said, "cancer is synonymous with chemo. I think my fear of chemo is greater than any fear of death. Chemo was such an awful experience—and I've had a double whammy since I've gone through it twice. Is it common to be so fearful of the chemo?"

"Well, fears of a recurrence are very common, but I'm not aware of the specific fear of chemotherapy." After a thoughtful pause, she said. "The person you should talk with is Dr. T., our psychologist. She would know much more about this. I'll call her to see if she can meet with you today."

We talked for another half hour about infertility, Shea, other effects, and my most recent cancer episode. When we'd finished, Melissa said, "Anything else I can do for you right now? Any other questions?"

"You've done a lot already," I said. "I'm so glad I got back in touch. I hope you'll keep me posted."

"You bet. That's what we're here for."

She called Dr. T, and we were in luck. Just one hallway over, we found a mental health professional devoted to helping childhood cancer survivors like me to manage the nagging worries. And the service was free! What a system!

After I sat in the chair across from Dr. T.'s desk and reeled off my fears of "*chemotus vomitus*," she offered a solution. "You know, chemo is quite different from when you were last treated. We now have very effective medications that *prevent* nausea. In fact, many patients don't experience nausea at all. If they do, it's much milder than you just described. We also have individual treatment rooms. How about a tour of this unit? Maybe seeing the new 1995 version of chemotherapy treatment will help allay your fears."

She escorted us down the hall. With still vivid memories of the old 1971 Torture Chamber, I felt like I was walking onto the set of a futuristic sci-fi movie. Only two child patients were receiving chemo, but each of them was nestled in his own room on his own La-Z-Boy recliner, watching TV and looking quite cozy. The IV was hooked up and dripping, but neither victim appeared sick, sad, or fatigued from vomiting. From the expressions on their faces, they were just having quiet time, as if they were resting up for an excursion to the mall.

I felt greatly relieved, though doubtful that two sightings would undo memories of fifty-six gut-wrenching chemo treatments. Still, it was a start. We walked out of St. Jude comforted to have restored our link to this storehouse of knowledge, yet frightened by the new clouds on my horizon.

When we returned to Nashville, I tried hard to keep life in focus. Yet the images flashing by gave me a bad case of psycho-vertigo. On the one hand, I marveled at the ease of my latest treatment. My chest was healing without complication. On the other hand, an emotional storm was brewing. The clouds of fear-ridden pollution were seeding my psyche with thoughts of betrayal, anger, and an inchoate sexual identity crisis.

For the previous seventeen years, I had dutifully subscribed to a lifestyle regimen that I believed gave me the upper hand over the cancer demons. I had minimized my stress, practiced yoga, enjoyed a wholesome vegetarian diet, and spent much of my time breathing pure country air. I had meditated and mentally visualized my way through the rough spots. I was Master of My Little Kingdom. Without realizing it, my confidence had grown to a delusional state. But now this third bout of cancer and the new information from St. Jude shattered my delusions. I felt betrayed— betrayed by myself *and* by both the alternative and mainstream medical establishments.

So I went to Burger King for a Whopper. The next week, I went to Wendy's for a quarter pounder, hold the cheese. Next, I ate four, three-inch-square, melt-in-your-mouth Krystal hamburgers. I tried every fast-food burger in town.

Screw it, I rationalized. *All those years lost to wheat berry casserole and tofu cheesecake, why did I go to the trouble? Why did I go out of my way to hike or swim? Why did I try to balance stress with plenty of rest and a regular practice of yoga? What difference did it make?*

My disdain for the pharmaceutical industry was also reaching a feverish pitch. Estrogen was the source of my vitriol, or more accurately, the manufacturers of the hormone replacement therapy I'd taken after my ovaries were removed. Although suspicions about artificial hormones had infiltrated my worry zone for more than a decade, I had never attempted to dissect my nebulous assumptions. With the loss of a breast and possibly more to come, I began to construct a more rational set of HRT factoids that invigorated my anger toward the makers of this ubiquitous drug.

At the time, questioning the value of this wonder cure was heresy. But as the supporting evidence rolled in, I felt more convinced that HRT and its manufacturers had played a role in promoting the growth of my breast cancer. My doctors had *not* maliciously misled me. They'd misled themselves. Overwhelmed by HRT proponents in the face of a huge problem, they'd misplaced their critical thinking skills.

The evidence had been right before their Hippocratic eyes. If tamoxifen *decreased* the risk of breast cancer by suppressing the action of estrogen, wouldn't it make sense that adding estrogen could *increase* the risk? If estrogen did not play a role, why was *every* breast cancer patient tested to determine whether her tissue responded to estrogen? And should millions of women be encouraged to take a medication which might increase their risk of the most prevalent form of cancer in women?

Some years later, the risks versus benefits of HRT for women at risk for breast cancer became a hotly debated issue, and after its purported cardiovascular benefits were invalidated, its use dropped dramatically. Some public health experts have speculated this decrease in use may be the primary reason behind the decrease in breast cancer incidence. The debate is ongoing, with some recommending short-term use when quality of life is greatly affected.

At that time, though, I still needed to learn more about HRT, so I arranged a consultation with Seth Cooper. Unfortunately, I put him on the defensive when I asked, "Why didn't you tell me I was at such high risk for breast cancer?"

Seth seemed unnerved by my question, which unnerved me as well. I hadn't intended to insult him. He had been my physician for more over sixteen years, and I'd always felt comfortable initiating an honest discussion, confident his response would be rooted in his devotion to my best interests. But when I posed this question, I was shocked to see his warm, relaxed demeanor transform into the steely armor of a robo-doc.

"The studies about increased breast cancer risks for long-term survivors like you just started coming out recently." His rigid posture and defensive tone clearly communicated, *I'm feeling mighty uncomfortable.*

To this day I'm not sure what caused his discomfort. In truth, I greatly admired this man. He had repeatedly gone far beyond other physicians, spending hours patiently explaining my body's latest shenanigans and the options for follow-up. Yet in my emotionally stressed state, I felt he bore some responsibility for not recognizing and informing me of the degree of my risk, and perhaps I had unconsciously assaulted him.

After that, I took a different tack. "Do you think the estrogen I was taking had anything to do with my breast cancer?"

Without revealing my peppery attitude toward HRT, I tried to engage Seth in a discussion about the possible role of supplemental estrogen in promoting breast cancer. He was not buying it. Even my first-person story about the strangely coincidental disappearing-reappearing act of my lump coinciding with the off-again, on-again consumption of the estrogen did not sway him.

He did not totally deny the correlation, but his sentiment was, "I look at the evidence and weigh the risks versus the benefits. HRT offers numerous benefits for two of the most likely causes of morbidity for women—heart disease and osteoporosis—and to my knowledge, the risks of breast cancer are minimal. And since you have not been producing sufficient estrogen for years, your risk of osteoporosis is a significant concern. So I can only conclude this medication is warranted for many women, including you."

I left Seth's office and swung by Rotier's, a local diner, to check out one of their award-winning hamburgers. The hunk of beef, medium well, served on toasted French bread and sucked down with fat-laden fries, was just what I needed to soothe my soul.

Seth was not alone in his commitment to HRT's virtues. None of the other excellent physicians I talked with was willing, ready, or able to put two and two together to acknowledge HRT might increase the risk of breast cancer. None was ready to admit that someone like me, who was already at an increased risk, maybe, just maybe, should not have taken the HRT.

These dedicated physicians stuck by their original recommendation for supplemental hormones. I believe their blindness arose from three overriding factors: (1) relentless advertising on the life-saving benefits of HRT for those poor, pitiful postmenopausal women struggling with hot flashes and mood swings; (2) lack of motivation to explore alternatives; and (3) willingness to substitute blanket recommendations for *individualized* care, regardless of the degree of individual risk. Groupthink fueled by pharmaceutical marketing trumped commonsense.

And so it goes. The same message bombarded millions of women: *If you have hot flashes, you need HRT! It will not only cure sizzling hot flashes, it will also help keep your bones strong and prevent the leading cause of death— heart disease! It may even keep your mind sharp and help prevent Alzheimer's disease! You would be a fool to pass up this miracle drug!*

I was one of those women who'd succumbed to the pitch.

But now the picture of my future relationship with the HRT pushers and their product was coming into focus. What was done was done. If I wanted to continue receiving medical care from first-rate doctors, unconstrained by fears of malpractice suits or verbal assaults from kooks like me, I had to keep my opinions to myself.

1996

As we slid our way into 1996, Barry, Shea and I resumed a fairly regular schedule. With Shea now in the fourth grade, I juggled work, chauffeuring her to school, piano lessons, and sleepovers with her inseparable friend, Savannah, while squeezing in a yoga class or night out with Barry. The easy challenge of my role as national coordinator of a controversial program pitting public health advocates against the multinational infant formula industries, the American Hospital Association and the US Department of Health and Human Services, was a much-needed distraction. The irony of the rabid one-breasted Amazon Mama taking on this triumvirate for the protection of the breast's divine purpose was lost on most.

Nevertheless, toward the end of January, the abundant love of my family and friends could not hold back a deepening depression stemming from my unsettling androgynous self-image. My singular-breasted chest deflated my sense of femininity, and my sex drive, already weakened from surgery, plummeted farther.

The coming out party of the sexually confused Minda occurred in January when my Perfect Ten women's group gathered for a hot tub party at Kathleen's home. Although I had revealed my wound like a badge of courage to several friends, this was more public. Sliding into a hot tub, baring all amidst these attractive women, was my first true act of confession that I was permanently maimed.

Humans are such a weird species. The New Guinea bird of paradise (the bird, not the flower) primps and prances to attract a mate for one purpose only — to keep the species alive. The *Homo sapiens* female, on the other hand, works hard at looking sexy long after her reproductive years have passed, to feed her ego as much as to attract a companion. If I'm not mistaken, neither purpose does much to help our species thrive. So there I was, sitting in a hot tub, with no ovaries, no eggs, only one breast, and no representatives of the opposite sex in sight. Yet my voracious ego still needed to believe I was sexually provocative.

My dear friends rallied with a performance worthy of a Golden Globe. "Minda," Debbie said, "you are still a stunningly beautiful woman. And it's not just your physical beauty. It's your strength, your courage, your ability to weather storm after storm. You are an inspiration to us all, with or without your breast."

They all nodded, and their sugar-coated feedback served as a much-needed support to my faltering self-worth. Soon we moved on to the forty-leventh discussion of how to restructure our group to deal with its varied personalities.

Separating myself from the common joys of my gender left me hanging in colorless territory. I wasn't gay, so I did not have to go through the unfathomable stress of a true coming out. However, I found myself in gender purgatory, devoid of the usual inclinations such as interest in grooming and motivation to flirt. Apparently the effective dosage for an active sense of sexiness was two matching breasts.

Still, this androgynous Minda mellowed into her new image rather quickly. (I'm not sure Barry has ever adapted, although he stoically accepted the situation.) Losing the sense of self-worth so closely linked to a hunk of fat and withered glands led to an awakening of a dormant source of freedom. I had invested a ridiculous amount of energy into winning some small sign of positive feedback when a member of the male species walked into the room. I was happily married, so what I needed that reassurance for, I'm not sure. What do we women do with that information? But once the expectation was gone, I became a liberated woman, and the freed energy buoyed my spirits in ways I had never experienced.

It wasn't long, though, before the boundaries of my liberation were put to the test.

chapter nine

1997

Just as I was getting comfy in the skin of androgynous Minda, my body began to suffer the consequences of its lopsided terrain. My discarded C-sized boob had weighed about the same as a large red Delicious apple. When the apple was picked off the tree, the branch popped up a couple of inches. As a result, my right shoulder rested higher than the left. Try walking around with your shoulders out of alignment day after day. My muscles began to feel bruised and contorted. With the unbalanced weight distribution and the accompanying achiness, I became a single-mounded malcontent.

So I went to see the fake-boob lady. A fake detachable breast, better known as a prosthesis, was obtained like contraband—in a private, low-lit room where no one else could observe the transaction between dealer and user. The professionals who sold these goods hocked their wares in the backs of lingerie stores, behind the racks of lacey underpants, push-up bras, and slinky nightgowns. According to the prosthesis pimps, Rebecka Vaughan Lingerie was the preferred dealer.

I slipped through the shop's front door, sneaked up to the cash register and whispered to the woman behind the counter, "I'd like to see someone about getting fitted for a prosthesis."

"Oh, yes," she quickly replied. With a sly glance, she called out softly across the display floor, "Mrs. Clarke, there's someone here to see you."

A matronly woman with a spray-stiffened gray pompadour approached me. "May I help you?" She seemed to be waiting for me to give her the password.

I felt an urge to murmur, *Max Smart here. The bridge has been flattened.* This was dangerous business, though, requiring the utmost caution. So I played it straight. "I've had a mastectomy and would like to get a prosthesis."

"Come on back," she said, and Bingo! I was in.

She turned about-face and walked to the dressing room without looking back, knowing I would follow. We slipped through the double curtains into a closet-sized space with barely enough room for the two of us.

"I'm so sorry you've had breast cancer, but we're going to get you fixed up. How long ago did you have surgery?"

"It's been a few months. A Reach to Recovery volunteer gave me a bra with stuffing that I thought would be sufficient, but it's not doing the job. There's some soreness because my shoulders seem out of alignment."

"A prosthesis should definitely help. We'll fix you up. Remove your blouse and your bra, and let me take a look."

I dared not disobey her orders. Once I'd disrobed, she stepped back, folding her arms across her chest in a posture of authority. She stared at my bare chest, sizing me up to estimate the quantity of goods I might need. After a few long, awkward seconds (for me), she said, "I'll be right back."

I stood topless in the dressing room, mulling over the scene. *It's amazing the hoops women will jump through to get mounds sitting pretty on their chests.*

I looked in the mirror at my Amazon warrior chest. It really didn't look so dreadful. In fact, the bare, one-breasted chest was not as unseemly as the clothed one-breasted chest. The bare chest said, "I am strong woman—hunter, gatherer, protector, goddess." The clothed chest said, "I am weak and maimed. Ignore me." In that moment, I accepted the fact that I was not totally liberated after all. I still needed two mounds to complete my outer self.

Mrs. Clarke walked in and said, "Here we are!"

She held in her hand a rubbery, satiny smooth, flesh-colored blob. She handed it to me to coddle. The silicone blob was slightly cold, but felt sumptuous in my hand. I had a strong impulse to squeeze it, slowly, again and again, like a ball of bread dough. I held it up by the top edge and placed it against my flattened chest where my vanished buddy had resided. It matched the real thing on the left almost exactly, having just the right degree of fullness and forty-year-old droop. Mrs. Clarke obviously had a black belt in fake-boob fitting. With just a few seconds of staring and without even asking my bra size, she had sized me up perfectly. I was in awe.

"Let's put it inside your bra and see how it fits."

I handed her my bra. It was one of those nifty numbers with a pocket in the cup for pillow stuffing, given to me by the American Cancer Society's Reach to Recovery program. She tucked the prosthesis in place.

"Now put this on," she instructed.

Without hesitation I loaded the saddle onto the horse. She leveled the two sides by digging her hands under the right, and then the left bra strap and adjusting each side accordingly. Her tugging and pulling on my intimate underwear and body parts seemed as natural as if she were my mother lovingly buttoning up my coat to send me off to school.

I put my blouse back on. Sure enough, both sides matched perfectly in size, shape, and alignment. You couldn't tell which one was the impostor. The density of the prosthesis balanced the weighty cargo of the authentic model on the left side, massaging my wounded chest, which squealed with joy.

"Thank you so much," I said. "Coming here felt a bit awkward, but now that I see how well you've matched my other breast, and how good it feels, I'm excited! No wonder so many people referred me here. Thank you!"

"It's something else, isn't it?" she modestly replied. "I've been in this business over twenty years, and they've really made a lot of progress with the designs. There used to be just a handful of shapes and sizes to choose from, but now there are dozens. It really is a boost for women just having gone through breast cancer."

"Yes it is," I agreed. "What an important service you provide!"

"They've made progress with the bras, too," she said. "Would you like to see a couple of our newer bras?"

"Sure." I sensed her coming sales pitch but was helpless to resist.

"What kind of bra do you usually wear?" she asked.

With this stranger, I launched into a kinky discussion of wires, lace, and fasteners. Do I like my breasts to stand up and out, Madonna-style pointy, or rounded and more natural? Do I prefer the fasteners in the back or front? Do I like a little lace showing through my blouse, or do I want the world to presume I wear no bra and that my forty-something breasts are extraordinarily firm enough to stay in the right place all by themselves?

Of course, I immediately knew the answers to all of these questions. I'd spent twenty-five years searching for just the right bra with just the right look and level of comfort. The long, hard-earned discovery of the Warner's Not-All-That-Bra®, Style 1058, size 34C, now had to be ditched for another model.

No need to fret. I was in the hands of an expert. She disappeared and returned a few minutes later with a few lovely specimens for my consideration. None were like my Not-All-That-Bra®, not even a distant cousin, so I had to resign myself to the knowledge that I had entered a new era of chest presentation and adornment.

These bras for the bosom-disabled came with a pocket inside each cup for the prosthesis. When the blob was inserted, it settled into place like its neighbor an inch away. Once the bra was hooked up and covered with clothing, not even the most experienced of boob watchers would be able to distinguish the difference. The pocketed blob felt luxurious against my chest, as if it belonged there.

I tried on two more bra models and settled on the least frilly of the three.

"There is one more thing," Mrs. Clarke said. "Younger women your age like this feature."

Her words reminded me that forty years old is young in breast cancer years.

She said, "You can order the prosthesis with an adhesive Velcro patch on the back that allows you to attach it directly to your chest, so you can go braless— in case you want to wear a strapless dress. Let me show you how it works."

She pulled out a three-inch-wide piece of flesh-toned fabric shaped like a small boomerang. She turned it over to show me how a thin layer of clear backing could be pulled off to expose a sticky layer that adheres to the skin.

She explained, "You attach the patch to your chest. Then attach the prosthesis with the Velcro backing to the patch."

Voila! Look, Ma, no bra!

"I can't believe this!" I said. "I'll take the whole package—the bra, the prosthesis, and the patches." I handed her my prescription. There actually was a prescription for this stuff.

"Follow me," she ordered, and we headed back through the curtains to the cashier's counter in the showroom. She went straight to the cash register, while I rifled through the nightgowns, trying not to blow my disguise as an ordinary customer fully loaded with two matching hunks of fat, ducts, and glands. I was just there like everyone else to purchase a seductive nightgown.

Mrs. Clarke looked up from the cash register. "Here we are, Ms. Lazarov."

I walked over to the counter to pay up. "You've got to be kidding!" I exclaimed.

The lump of silicone cost three hundred smackeroos! And that did not include the pocket bra or self-adhesive boomerangs. The blob was very nicely shaped, I admit, and was going to be fun to squeeze, particularly when I was under stress, but it probably did not cost much more to make than a Wham-O Super Ball®, which sold for $3.99. I wondered if the blob of silicone would bounce. Super Balls® at least bounced.

"That's what they cost," she said. "Your insurance will reimburse you, of course."

I was shocked. Her response jolted me back to the reality of corporate medicine. Oh, yeah, in case I'd forgotten, the economics of supply and demand was the basis on which our country thrived. *We supply what you want, so cough up whatever we demand. Your insurance is paying for it anyway, so what are you complaining about?*

In reverence to the holiness of the insurance provider's well-being, I swapped the equivalent of a month's grocery money for a blob of well-shaped silicone and a blob holster. I must confess, I left Rebecka Vaughan's a *very* happy customer.

Over the next couple of months, I began to experience both the joys and hassles of life with a detachable blob. First and foremost, when the blob was nestled into its pocket and hugging my chest, it felt marvelous! The right side of my bra no longer inched up my chest, and my shoulders were no longer tugged in all the wrong directions. When I plopped in the heavy blob, serenity reigned.

The blob also placed a constant, pleasant pressure on my wounded chest, similar to the healing touch of fingers on a headachy forehead. The blob's gentle, but firm pressure against the outside of my chest provided therapy for the sore, sometimes aching chest wall. The stick-on Velcro blob was also a precious innovation, allowing me to slip on a sexy persona with a braless dress or blouse. But then I discovered the downsides of a detachable blob.

On a business trip to San Diego, I felt quite peppy and took an afternoon off to explore the picturesque seaside town of La Jolla. My ultimate goal was a swim in the ocean, so I headed to the public dressing room to change into my bathing suit. I began pulling the paraphernalia out of my backpack—lotion, towel, swimsuit, and boomerang. Oops. I had forgotten to bring the boomerang to attach the blob to my chest.

Moment of truth. Was I humble enough to display a one-breasted chest to these strangers? My haggard ego won out again, and I dropped the blob into the skimpy, stretched out, bra-like pouch inside my Speedo tank suit. The suit was not prosthesis-friendly. Its bra pouches were intended for mounds well anchored to the body. All the same, when I came out of the dressing room and paused in front of the bathroom mirror, I thought I looked pretty damn good, certainly good enough to parade down the hill to the beach with my chest held high.

I wasted no time submerging myself in the ocean. Within a minute, my smugness evaporated. The blob slipped out of place and dropped down into the crotch of my bathing suit. I scanned my surroundings. Thankfully, no one had spotted my migrating bulge, so I felt safe to start digging around inside my suit. I stooped down so only my head poked above the water, reached down into the one-piece suit, and snatched the wayward blob from my crotch. Again I stood up, looked around, then slid under the water and dropped the blob back into my swimsuit bra. Realizing there was no way to hold the blob in place for long, I crossed my arms against my chest pretending I was cold, waded out of the water, and returned to the dressing room.

The short ocean dip at La Jolla was over, along with my free-wheeling tendencies toward spontaneous side trips, which at the present were severely hampered by the absence of a three-inch piece of Velcro. Frustrated, I got dressed, gathered my things, and headed to the bus stop to catch a ride back to San Diego. I never left home again without the boomerang—until the novelty wore thin.

Another downside was the time limit. The manufacturers of the stick-on blob understood a glue strong enough to defy the gravity of a half-pound hunk of silicone might be irritating to the skin, so the boomerangs came with a small bottle of goo to be applied to the skin prior to attaching the blob. Unfortunately, the irritation-prevention goo also weakened the effect of the adhesive. Once the goo, boomerang, and blob were attached, the clock started ticking. I had about three hours before I turned into a one-mounded pumpkin.

One night I was sitting in a restaurant, having dinner with the gals, immersed in conversation, sipping on my second glass of wine and enjoying my *crème brûlée*, when I felt the blob disengaging itself from my chest.

As if nothing was happening, I casually rose from my chair. "I'll be back in a minute."

Once out of sight, I dashed to the restroom. Inside the stall, I inspected the damage. I was lucky. The boomerang and blob were only one-third detached, so I had a few more minutes before my cover of coolness became completely unglued.

I returned to the table. "I'm really tired, ladies. I think I'm going to head home."

By the time I got to the car, the blob was barely hanging on. I looked around the parking lot to make sure I was alone. Once I was in the driver's seat, I reached down into my shirt and ripped off the dangling blob and boomerang. Aaahhh.

These awkward incidents, in addition to an irritating rash from the adhesive, created a growing awareness of the absurdity of my desire for a stick-on blob. I eventually came to my senses and gave up on the braless look.

As winter deferred to spring, I adjusted to my new state of mind and body. My longstanding effort to eat plenty of whole grains, fruits, and veggies was replaced by a new, subconscious revolt to abandon the cornerstones of my lifestyle and eat anything I damn well pleased. I even considered taking up cigarettes (not seriously). Occasionally, I substituted a Whopper for my tofu salad sandwich, and more and more frequently, I reached for a bag of BBQ Fritos instead of a peach.

Then Vicki dropped into my life again. Vicki was a friend and former colleague employed as a nutritionist for a National Cancer Institute study in San Diego. She heard through the grapevine of my most recent cancer battle and called to offer her love and condolences. During the conversation, she filled me in on her current work. She and her colleagues were investigating the impact of large quantities of fruits and vegetables on the prevention of a variety of cancers. I lamented about my latest misadventures in healthy eating.

"Minda," she said, "do you realize how many studies have been published demonstrating the strong correlation between the consumption of fruits and veggies and a decreased prevalence of several cancers? It's astounding."

We chatted for a long time while she described the new data on how dozens of naturally occurring chemicals in fruits and vegetables aided the prevention of lung, colon and other cancers. Phytochemicals, she called them.

"Let me send you some information. How about a few recipes, too?" she asked.

The conversation with Vicki helped me reconnect with the wisdom of my previous tenets for good health. Although I was still skeptical whether a wholesome lifestyle could prevent cancer, my eyes had been reopened to the possibility.

Vicki sent me recipes for carrot-beet-celery-tomato juice, carrot-pumpkin bread, and winter squash soup. She said the goal was to consume twelve servings every day of high-octane fruits and veggies loaded with phytochemicals. I made a gallant attempt to follow the protocol. Unfortunately, discipline was not one of my strengths. I fared better following my own roundabout way, so by the end of the second week, I was feeling pretty proud of myself if I had cantaloupe for breakfast, a sweet potato for lunch, and a spinach enchilada for dinner.

I scored better in doing my own research to learn more about the relationship between fruits, veggies and cancer. I had taken on an additional gig as a nutrition instructor at the Vanderbilt School of Nursing, so coming up with a new lecture on the role of nutrition in preventing cancer would be just the jump-start I needed. The breadth of information I uncovered astonished me. I found more than a hundred and twenty studies documenting this positive effect. Although most of the studies were largely epidemiologic and, therefore, not intended to prove direct cause and effect, the evidence was compelling. Government trials like the one Vicki was working with would generate invaluable evidence.

I felt like an idiot. Here I was, a reasonably intelligent master's level nutritionist, and I'd been oblivious to the immense and growing body of data showing the importance of scarfing down as many fruits and veggies as possible. Five a day. I knew the shtick and tried to practice it, but I rarely succeeded. In preparation for the lecture, I also studied the more recent theories on *how* cancer gets started and what stimulates its growth once the seeds are planted.

With this new knowledge, I struck a much-needed balance between the possibilities for *and* the limitations of control. Prior to the breast cancer, I felt in total control. After the diagnosis, I felt no control. Now my fulcrum was right in the middle. Balance—that essential, but elusive equilibrium—helped me reclaim the sound rationale that I *could* do something to help myself.

On the one hand, I did not have to sit back and let the cancer demons plow right through my body. Yet on the other hand, I no longer felt the full responsibility, and thus the guilt, of not doing enough. What a relief. The responsibility of commandeering all the troops all the time was much too tiresome!

My new and improved outlook shifted my psyche, my spirit, and my demeanor to a much healthier vantage point. Life reached a normalcy with work, family, and friends once again fulfilling my days. Meetings, presentations, and hospital visits for work, among other necessities like yoga classes and Shea's school and sports activities, consumed my attention as life eased back into the safe and familiar.

By August, 1997, my work with the Baby Friendly Program had evolved into a level of intensity demanding more than my battered body could bear, so I resigned from a twenty-year career in public health to take a sixteen-month sabbatical. My goal was to relax, garden, breathe the country air, eat more veggies, and help Shea prepare for becoming a Bat Mitzvah. The stage was set for a fabulous break.

Then, out of the insidious blind spot where danger always looms, came the Year from Hell: 1998.

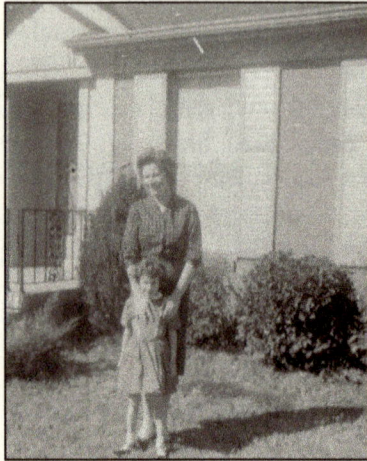

Minda and her mother, Matilda, 1961.

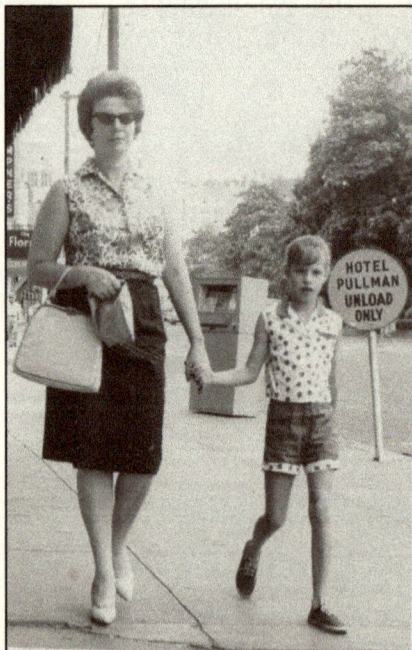

Matilda and Minda, 1964.

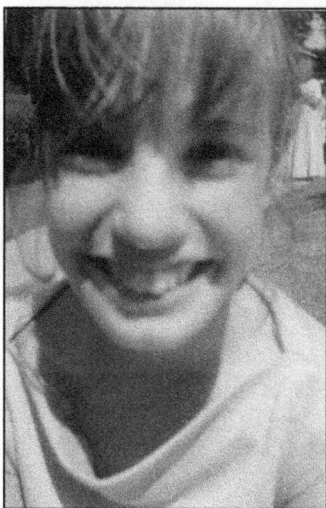

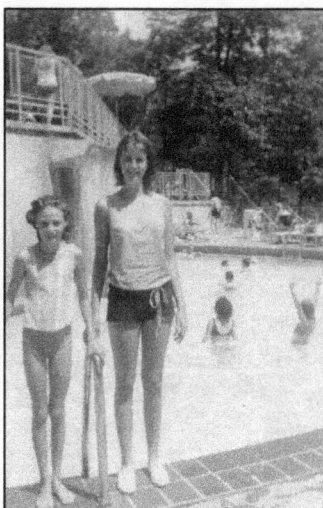

Minda (left); Minda and her sister, Reva (right),
in Hot Springs, Arkansas, summer 1965.

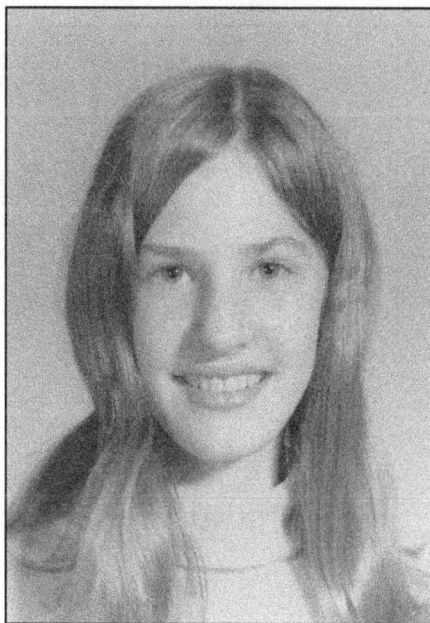

Minda's school photo, 1968.

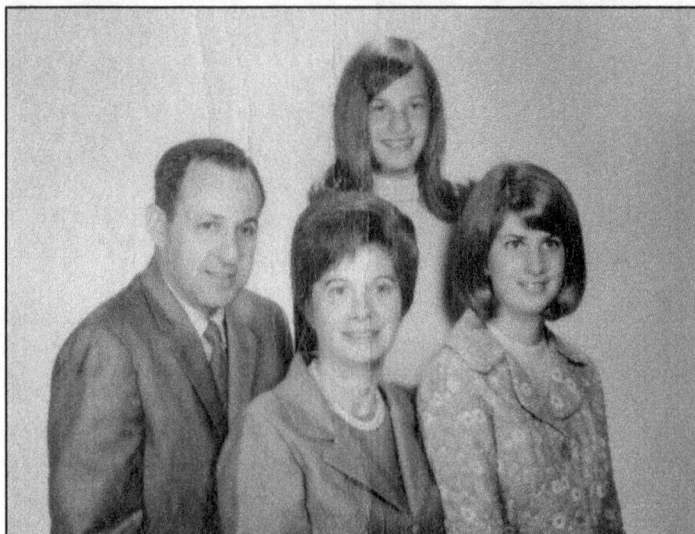

Israel, Matilda, Minda and Reva, 1968.

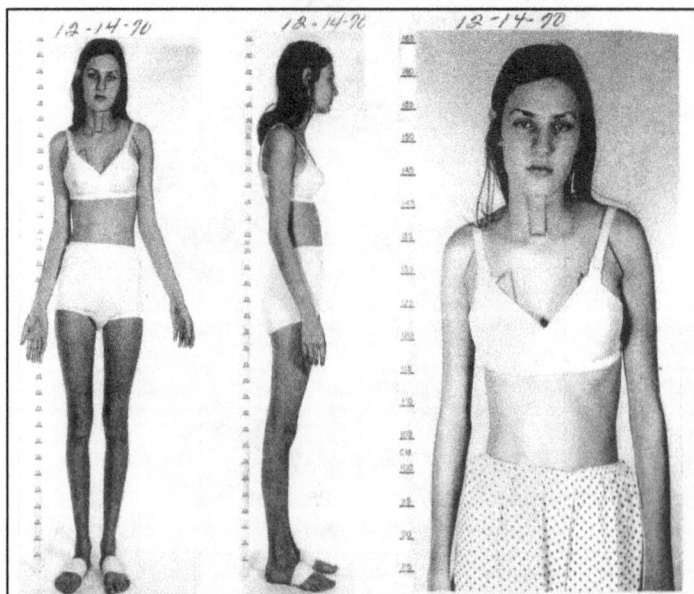

St. Jude Hospital photos of Minda, 1970.

St. Jude Highlights:

- Founded by Danny Thomas in 1962, the hospital, though named for St. Jude, is fully non-sectarian in nature. From the very start, children of all races, all religions were cared for—free.

- St. Jude's admits those children who are referred by doctors, and who suffer from one of the several catastrophic children's diseases it has under study.

- Leukemia was one of the first diseases to be chosen for concentrated attack at St. Jude's. At the time, it was incurable—a dread, fatal disease which is still America's leading child killer.

- Other forms of childhood cancer are also being intensely researched.

- Soon after the hospital was founded, St. Jude doctors found a way, through "massive therapy," to force all leukemia symptoms into remission. Chemotherapy and radiation are used to save a very high percentage of children from early death. Then, the problem is to keep them in remission, free of all symptoms.

- This can be done, successfully in about half of all cases, in out-patient treatment. Thus, thousands of children in all parts of the United States, living at home once again, depend for their lives upon regular visits back to the hospital—or to their own family doctor, who works with St. Jude's and uses drugs supplied free by St. Jude's.

- In 1971, newspapers, television, and many medical journals carried this exciting news: Dr. Donald Pinkel, medical director of the hospital, said, "Leukemia can no longer be considered an incurable disease." Now, more than 50% can attain a 5-year cure rate at St. Jude's. Other hospitals are adopting the treatment developed at St. Jude's; and this year three new medical textbooks are teaching the method.

- More children than ever are being brought to St. Jude's for care. A new seven-story addition will soon be erected—even though only half the money for it is yet available.

- Besides the millions of dollars needed to help pay for the addition, St. Jude's must raise more than $5,000,000 every single year for research and patient care!

- The battle is only half-won against leukemia: nearly 50% of the children stricken with it still die at St. Jude's. The fight to save them—and the victims of other childhood cancers—must go on!

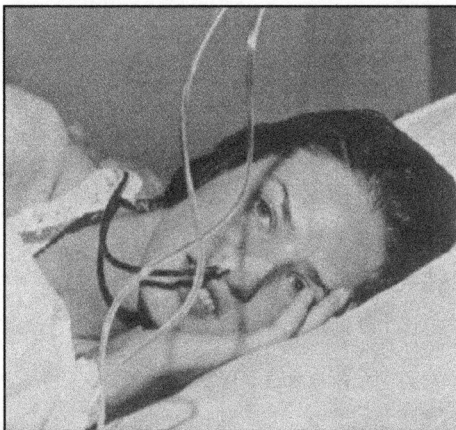

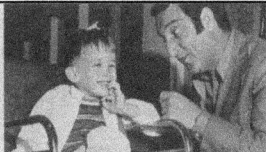

What it's all about . . .

CONTRIBUTIONS PAY TO KEEP THESE CHILDREN ALIVE!

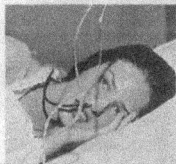

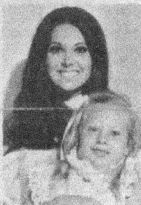

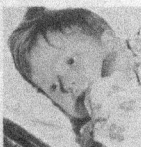

The newspaper clipping at the right was carried in papers all over the nation last spring.

This lovely little girl, as it happens, was not a patient at St. Jude's. But our patients die also —far too many of them.

To be sure, it is near-miraculous that we've reached a point where more than half can be saved. Our goal is to soon be able to give all stricken children a full and happy life.

We re-print this clip because this child's poem so dramatically illustrates just how much every boy and girl wants to cling to life—as is their right. We must help them; they can not help themselves.

Leukemia silences 'Thanks for Life'

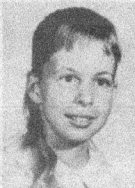

THANK-YOU FOR LIFE

Thank You Lord For Letting Me Be Alive Today
I Like To Try To Help In Many Ways.
Thank-You For My Family.
We Do Live Quite Happily.
We Always Play Together.
Oh! Thank-You For The Sunshine Weather.
IT'S JUST WONDERFUL TO BE ALIVE!

The parents of Tami Hogan, 9, who died last Thursday in Sacramento, Calif., of leukemia, have found this poem of hers. The girl was unaware she was dying when she wrote it. They ran across the poem with title, "Thank-You For Life," on the top page of her school work folder. They never had seen the poem before. (A.P.)

Minda in the St. Jude Appeal Letter, 1971.

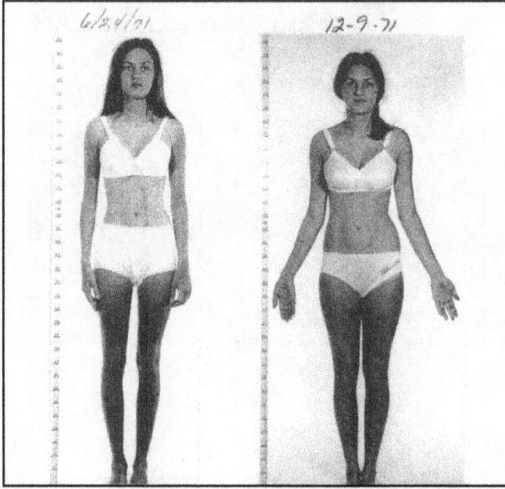

St. Jude Hospital photos of Minda, 1971.

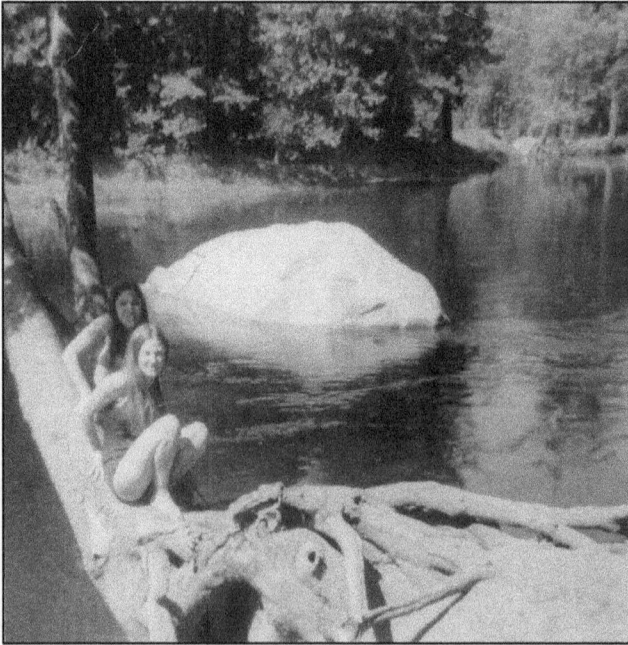

Minda and her best friend, Sharon Price,
in Yosemite National Park, 1972.

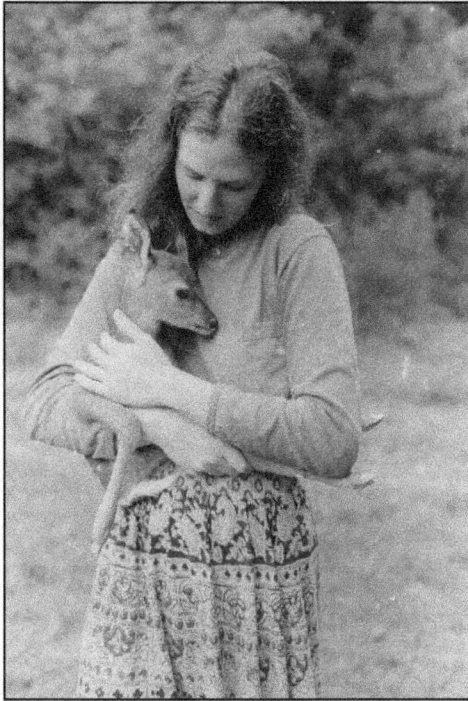

Top: Minda at home, summer 1979.

After rising from a post-treatment stupor, I took my usual therapeutic walk on the driveway. About ¼ mile into my cruise, I came upon what appeared to be an abandoned fawn — in a similar state of bewilderment that I was experiencing. Timid at first, she warmed right up to me following some gentle cuddling. Just as soon as I thought I had won her over, we heard a piercing cry of distress from the top of the hill. The fawn responded to her mother's call in a way we knew we couldn't deny. We took her to the top of the hill and let her go. I was sorry—not only to lose my new friend but also to realize I could not share her elevated spirits and energy...

Bottom: Minda's writing on the back of the above photo.

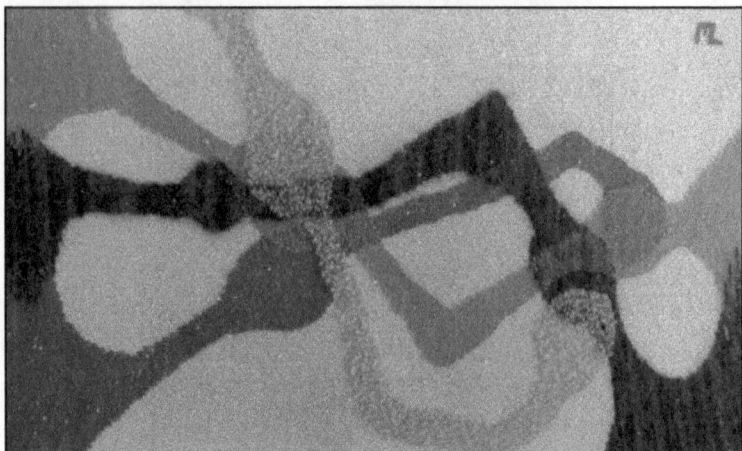

Minda took up weaving in the late seventies.
This weaving she titled "Woven Cancer", 1980.

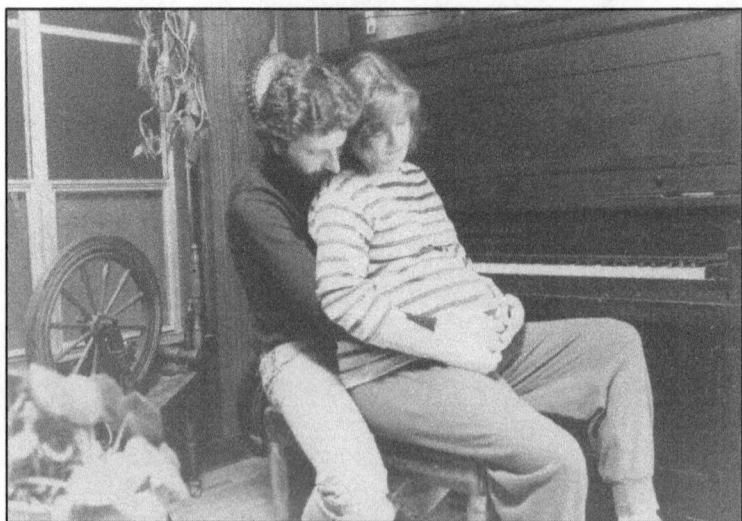

Minda pregnant with Shea, and her husband, Barry Sulkin,
at home in Nashville, 1985.

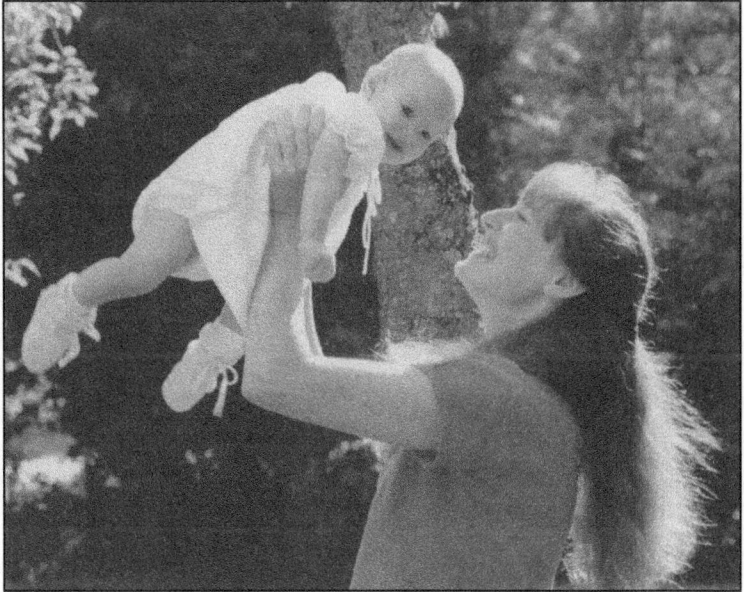

Minda holding her daughter, Shea, 1985.

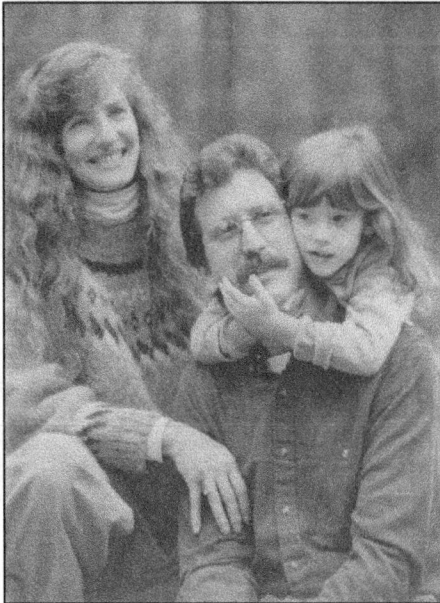

Minda, Barry and Shea, 1989.

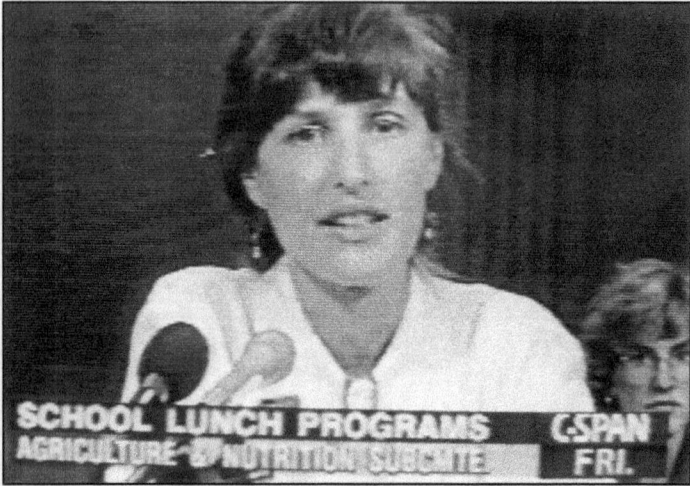

Minda testifying before Congress
advocating for increased support of breastfeeding
in the WIC (Women, Infants and Children) program, 1994.

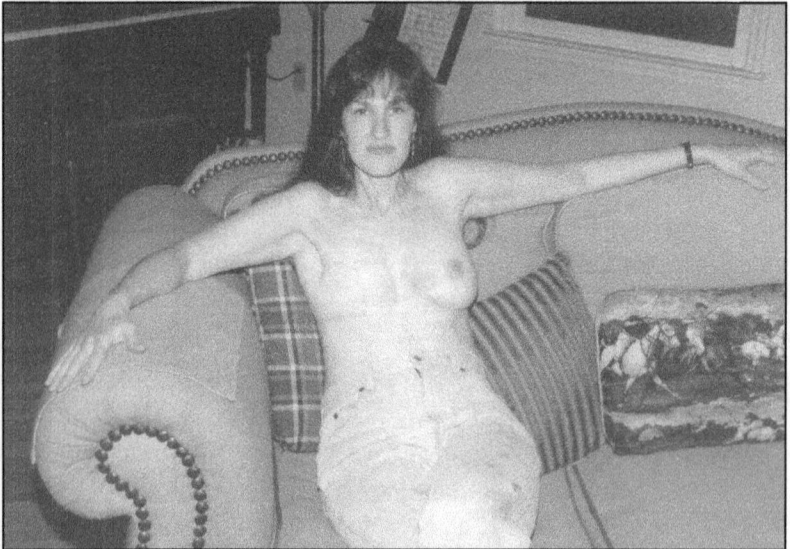

Minda at home in Nashville
just before her second mastectomy, 1998.

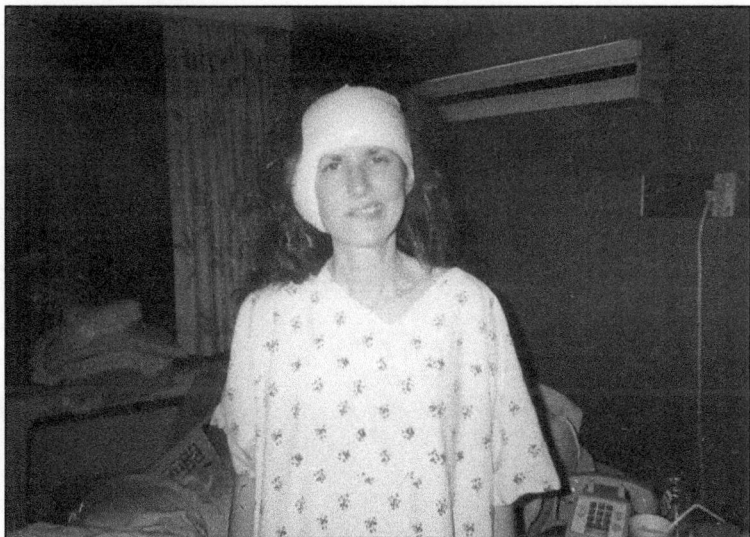

Minda in the hospital after acoustic neuroma surgery, 1998.

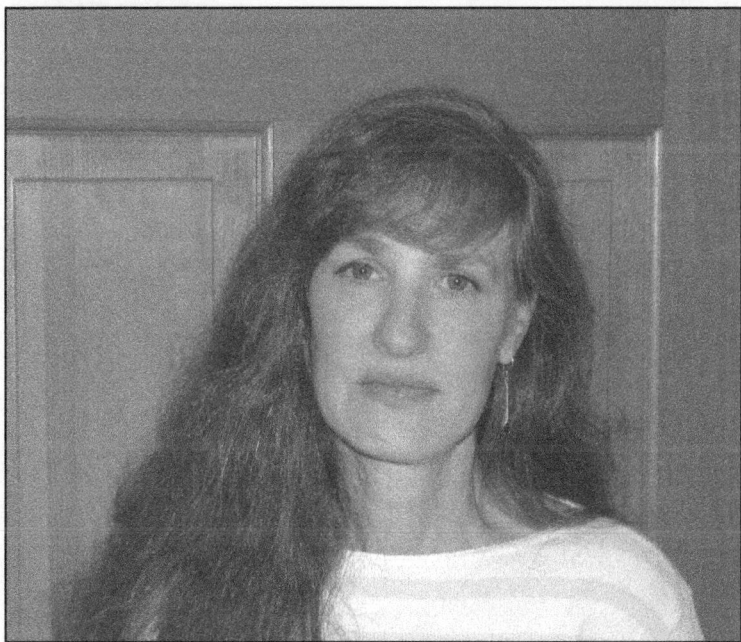

Minda, 2003.

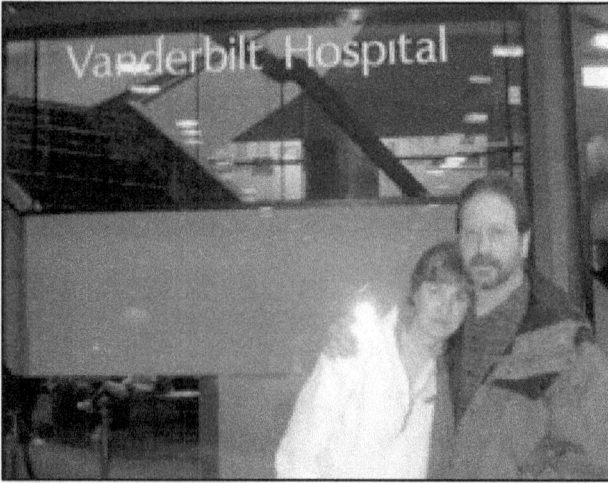

Minda and Barry before Minda's second brain surgery
for optic nerve tumor, 2006.

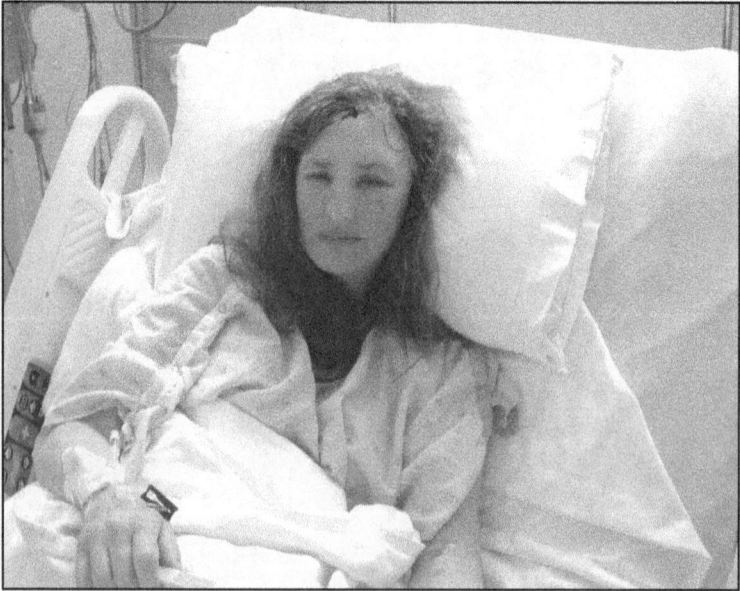

Minda in the hospital after optic nerve surgery, 2006.

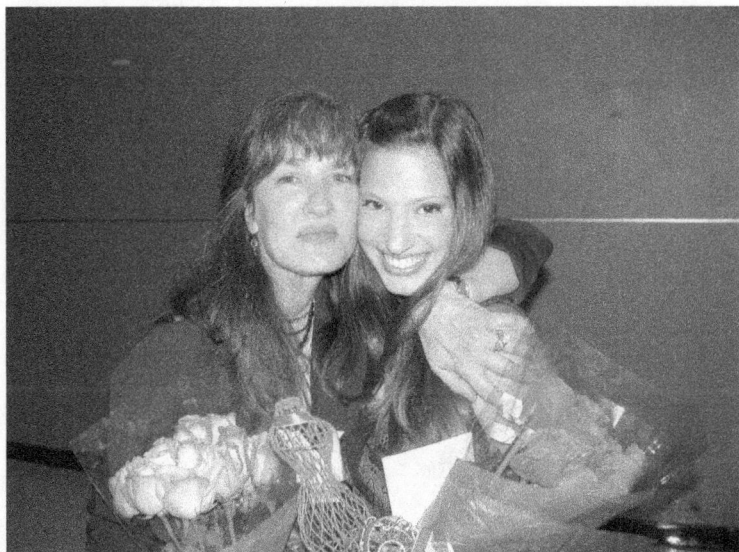

Minda with Shea, after Shea's undergraduate fashion show,
University of Texas, 2007.

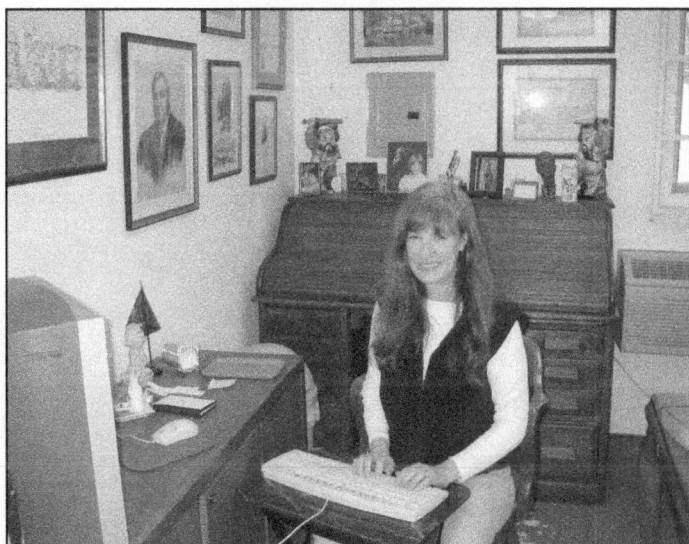

Minda working on this book
in her writing studio in a neighbor's barn, 2008.

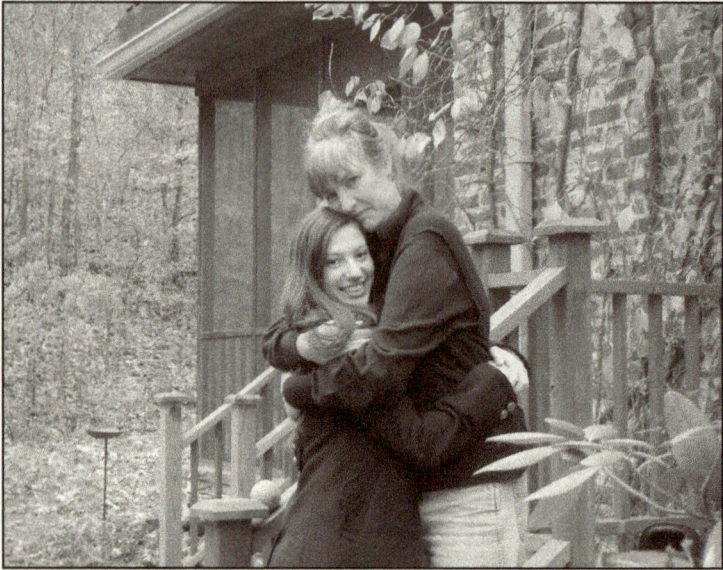

Shea visiting home during the time Minda was sick with
Epstein-Barr virus, 2008.

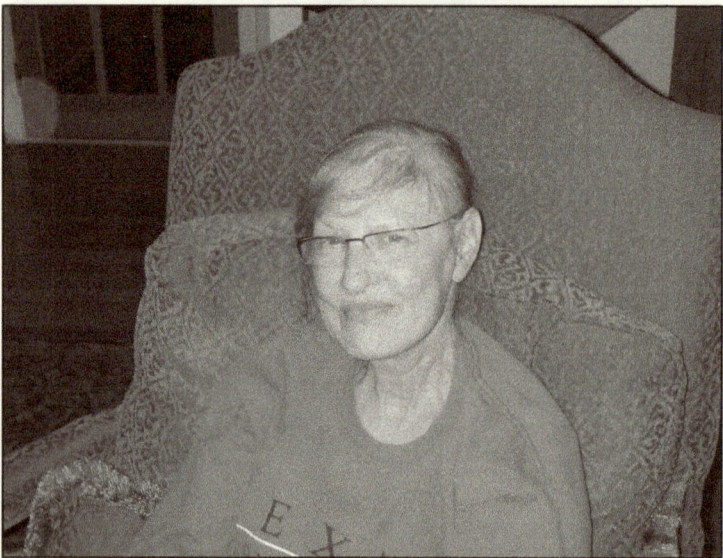

Minda during the months of chemo treatments, 2010.

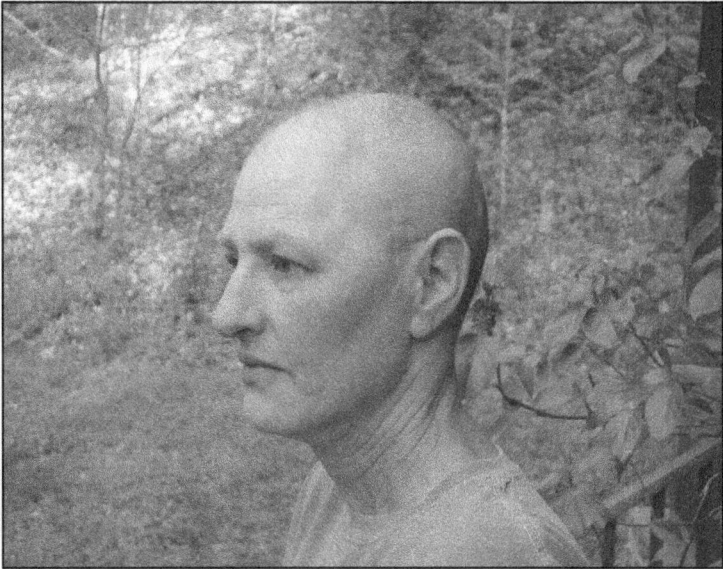

The first time Minda went bald from chemo, 2010.

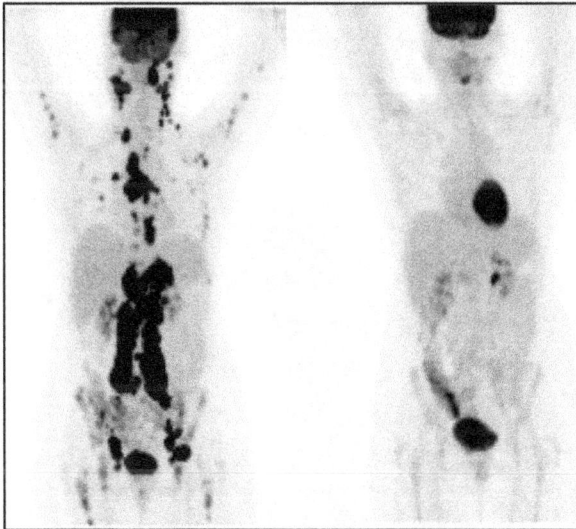

Left: PET scan of Minda, October 2009,
showing Epstein-Barr virus related B-cell Lymphoma.
Right: PET scan of Minda, January 2010,
after treatment showing no signs of Lymphoma.

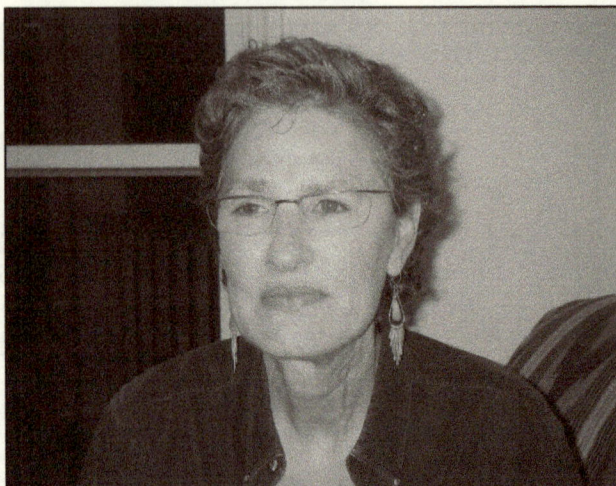

Minda, fall 2010.

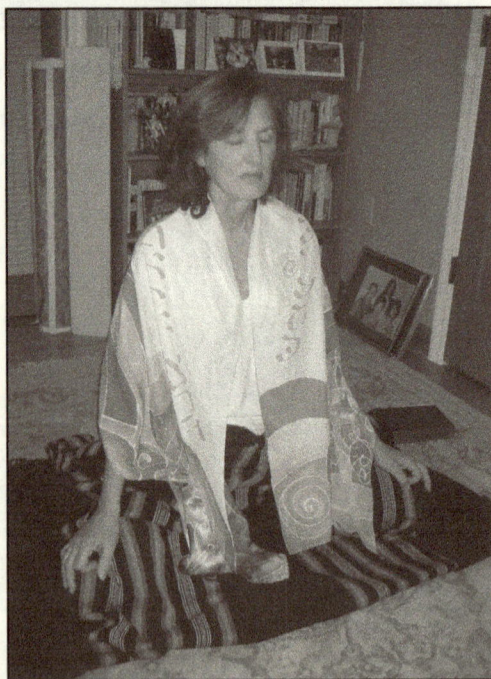

Minda practicing her daily meditation at home, August 2011.

chapter ten

1997, SEPTEMBER

Autumn was mammogram time. Following the breast cancer diagnosis in October, 1995, my lone breast nagged me for the annual portrait of her ducts and lobules. The portrait of 1996 was uneventful, so in the fall of 1997 when the leaves were peaking, I ignored my bosom buddy and talked myself into a detour. At the end of December, we were to celebrate my parents' fiftieth wedding anniversary in one of the most important traditions of my Jewish heritage—a family cruise to the Caribbean.

I strategically planned ahead and postponed the mammogram from October to mid-December, using the following logic: A mammogram would have one of two possible outcomes, negative or suspicious. The first scenario would, of course, be grand, and I could celebrate my parents' joyous occasion with a free spirit. The second scenario could be complicated. Suspicion would lead to a biopsy, which could lead to a mastectomy, which would lead to my absence or, worse, my possible impending demise and a dampening of the festive mood for all members of the family.

The best solution was to delay the mammogram until *after* the trip. No specific diagnosis, no Debbie Downer to interfere with the festivities. What difference could sixty days make?

Still, a pesky little voice kept badgering me about the lunacy of this delay. In order to appease it, I compromised a few days before the cruise and subjected the breast to the George Foreman Boobie Grill. This move would get the process started, but would not allow enough time for the follow-up that might unleash a cascade of worry. This fail-proof plan began to unravel after the first reading of the mammogram. I became wary when the technician called me back to redo the grilling. She was as cool and noncommittal as a confirmed bachelor. I allowed myself to be relieved by her lack of concern.

The next day I went to see Dr. Jeanne Ballinger for her interpretation of the radiologist's interpretation of the mammogram machine's interpretation. Not good, but not terrible was the message from Jeanne.

"There's a cyst and some new calcification in your left breast. The cyst I'm not worried about. The calcification is suspicious, however. It could be cancerous. If it is, it looks like the very early stages of what we call *ductal carcinoma in situ*. The cells are scattered—not even big enough to make a palpable mass."

"Oh." Pause.

She explained further. "*Ductal carcinoma* is the most common form of breast cancer. *In situ* means the cancerous cells are confined to the ducts, and we've hopefully caught it early."

"Mmmm." Pause. "This may sound like an odd request, but we're getting ready to go on a cruise to celebrate my parents' fiftieth anniversary. Can this wait until I get back?"

"Well, the next step is a stereotactic biopsy. Based on what I see from the pathologist's report, I don't see that it's important to do the biopsy before you leave."

We talked a bit more about a prophylactic mastectomy in the event the biopsy showed no cancer. Then I walked out, leaving my worries in the clinic room. In a distorted turn of events, I was feeling oddly relieved. From all vantage points, it seemed I was heading down a path of Bye-Bye to Bosom Buddy Number Two. I did not want to lose my good friend. At the same time, I did not mind the thought of ridding myself of the source of a worry always lightly perched on my shoulder and whispering, *When will the cancer demons launch their rockets into my left breast?*

So what might have been a nerve-racking bon voyage became a mildly restrained departure.

Seven days of jumping from island to island passed without a glitch, unless of course you consider the thirty-six hours without air-conditioning and my mother sick with the flu, stuck in her claustrophobic closet of a state room for almost the entire trip. I managed to mostly forget about the itty-bitty time bombs ticking away in the lining of my ducts.

1998

Three days after our return, I picked up where I'd left off and escorted my breast to the Baptist Women's Clinic for a stereotactic biopsy. I had no expectations of what this procedure would entail. The word *stereotactic* meant absolutely nothing to me. The little movie screen in my mind that usually ran the previews of the day's feature was blank. So maybe I should *not* have been shocked when they asked me to lie face-down on a table with one big hole for my breast to dangle through.

Ah, one more invention by someone who did not have mammary glands. George Foreman Boobie Grill, silicone gel bag, and now this slip-breast-through-hole-and-poke-it-with-needles table. What would they think of next? Isn't it about time to recruit a few female biomedical engineers?

While I lay on my belly, the technician shoved me here and there until my left breast hung perfectly centered through the hole, like a dart through the bull's-eye. Then in another ingenious maneuver, he elevated the table so the doctor wouldn't have to be a yogic master to get to my breast. For the "stereo" part of the procedure, the tech compressed my breast with a specialized mammography machine to obtain multiple computerized images. Next, the doc stepped up to give me a few little pricks of Novocaine, and I was good to go for the "tactic" part.

With the computerized images as a guide, the doctor inserted a needle into my breast. Additional images were taken at this point to assure the doctor had hit the targeted tissue. Similar to a core drill, he sucked out a skinny earthworm-like sample, then rotated the needle to get another sample. In under ten minutes, the doctor managed to suck, rotate, suck, rotate . . . (you get the idea) until he had all the samples he needed. Amazingly, I felt only a little pressure. When he lowered the table and let me get up, I got dressed and headed home.

Unlike the last confrontation with breast biopsies, I no longer naïvely expected the cancer demons to pass me by. This time around, I was not just *expecting* the worse. I had already accepted it. By the next day when I showed up for my appointment to discuss the results with Jeanne, there was no wiggle room for doubt.

Jeanne wasted no time. "Well, Minda. I'm sorry. It's cancer again."

"It's okay. Well, it's not okay, but you know what I mean."

"I know what you mean. Then again, I don't know what you mean since I haven't had cancer."

"I know exactly what you mean!"

We both laughed.

"As before, it looks like we caught this really early. The biopsies showed two grades of cancer in your breast. Both of them are different from the type of cancer you had before. The majority of the cancerous cells are the most common type and the least aggressive, the *ductal carcinoma in situ* that we talked about. Some of the tissue, however, is an intermediate-to-high grade invasive *ductal carcinoma*—a more aggressive type."

My mind was already running away to its safe numb shelter of shock. Even though I was expecting a fly ball, this had thrown me a curve, so away my mind retreated, unable to hear anything more. I managed to get through the rest of the conversation as she explained the mastectomy and reconstruction. When I left, I felt relieved and not relieved—if you know what I mean.

The saga of my irradiated breasts was coming to an end. Hundreds of rads of radiation to my budding teenage breasts, the equivalent of thousands of chest X-

rays, with a potent dessert of fifty-six CanceRid
treatments, had allowed the cancer demons to be
fruitful and multiply. They had found a tolerant home,
hunkered down and waited for twenty-seven years.
Had my low-fat, high-antioxidant diet held them in
check for a while? Had I never taken any estrogen,
would they have eventually pulled off their victory
anyway? Should I have taken tamoxifen to delay the
second breast cancer?

A scenario emerged that put all of these queries in
perspective and helped ease my growing anxiety. The
cancer in Bosom Buddy Number Two was caught so
early, there was no palpable lump. The cancer demons
were just beginning to organize their troops. Here's an
interesting thought: If I had shown up for the
mammogram a couple of months earlier when I was
supposed to, the cancerous cells might not have been
detectable.

In this scenario, many months or even a year might
have passed before a self-examination or the next
mammogram detected a lump—perhaps too late for the
higher grade invasive cancer to be controlled. B'shert!
My stupidity to delay the mammogram might have
saved my life.

Conjuring up this theory made me feel lucky. I'd
won the lottery—again! Now all I had to do was have
Bosom Buddy Number Two lopped off. And on top of
all this good fortune, I get to choose two new breasts!
What more could a girl ask?

A simple mastectomy was scheduled in two weeks.
"Simple" in this case was a euphemism for chopping off
the breast and only a few neighboring lymph nodes for
a "sentinel node biopsy." The muscle and other more
distant nodes would be left intact. Two weeks were just

enough time to figure out who I should trust to sculpt artificial breasts and what medium should be used for the artistry.

With two years' experience juggling a prosthesis, I no longer felt any doubt about sculpting or not sculpting. I was ready for mounds that would not crawl up my chest, drop down into my crotch, or reside on top of the dresser every night. So much for the freedom of Androgynous Minda.

I called Melissa at St. Jude to pluck the wisdom from her data-dense, commonsense brain. She was quick with her response. Simple mastectomy was a good idea. She also recommended I find a plastic surgeon specializing in irradiated chests.

"The radiation you had as a teenager affects the elasticity of the chest so it won't stretch very easily to allow room for the implants. It's important for you to find a surgeon who has experience working with patients who've had extensive radiation."

"Not a problem," I said. "Dr. Ballinger mentioned this to me when we discussed reconstruction. I don't envision big breasts anyway. I've already experienced the joys of big breasts, so I'm ready to downsize."

Jeanne suggested Dr. F. at Baptist Hospital, where she had surgical privileges. I knew of Dr. F. because he was the father of one of Shea's classmates. Nine days later, I was more than ready and willing for a consult with the plastic surgeon. My natural breasts had never matched each other. My slightly larger right breast had always hung a tad lower than my left. But now a matched set was in my future!

The nurse escorted me into the examining room, then spent an ample thirty minutes discussing the options. The three choices were the same as before: mound by implant, mound by transplanting a back muscle on top of the implant, and mound by moving abdominal fat.

Once I confirmed my choice for the simplest route of implants, she pulled two models out of a cabinet to show me. One model was filled with saline, the other with silicone. She balanced one blob in each outstretched hand as if she were weighing heads of lettuce.

"Would you like to hold them?" she asked.

"Sure."

She handed them to me, one at a time. They both felt good in my hand, squishy, but with a firm resistance. The silicone-filled model felt more like the real thing, a youthful version from a perky twenty-five-year-old. The saline-filled implant had a more solid, resistant feel, like a well-inflated rubber ball.

"The casings of both implants are made of a rubberlike silicone," she explained. "The difference is what's on the inside. The silicone implant gives a more natural look." She held the silicone mound up by the top edge. "See how it hangs. It keeps its shape while it still has a small droop to give it a more realistic look."

Silicone gel or saline? She presented my choice in a nonchalant tone reminiscent of a clerk at McDonald's asking, "Do you want diet or regular Coke with your value meal?"

The more accurate question would have been, "Do you prefer harmless salt water or potentially toxic polydimethylsiloxane?"

This same choice was presented to thousands of women each year, though many nurses and plastic surgeons appeared sheepish when suggesting silicone. Perhaps they felt the risks were unfounded, but I was not buying it. Only three people would see my chest with any regularity—myself, Barry, and Dr. Seth Cooper. The shape of my breasts would not affect the quality of care from Seth. Nor was Barry's love and devotion grounded in the degree of my droopiness. And I hoped my own inner strength and spirituality were not linked to any aspect of my boobs. With no tangible reason to accrue any more unnecessary risks in this already risk-laden body, I chose saline-filled bags.

"I've had enough trouble," I told the nurse without skipping a beat. "The last thing I need is silicone leaking in my chest. I want the saline implants."

A side note of interest: In doing the research for this book, I learned there are no FDA safety tests for saline implants in the event of a rupture. Only the manufacturers of the hazardous silicone gel or the newer alternative fillers must subject their product to the safety tests. Does that tell us something?

The nurse pressured me no further. She went on to explain the risk of hardening of the chest wall around both types of the implants." Some women experience significant scarring that leads to tightening of the chest wall around the implant," she explained. "Only a few of these women experience enough discomfort to warrant additional surgery. But it's another factor you may want to consider."

She moved on, describing the steps for transforming One-Breasted Amazon Mama to Bilaterally Symmetrical-Youthful Minda.

"Here's how the surgery will work. During the mastectomy, Dr. F. will be waiting nearby for a call, and when Dr. Ballinger is finished with the mastectomy, Dr. F. will step in and take over. First, he'll place what's known as an expander under the pectoral muscles—the long, thin muscles that lie right on top of your chest."

She pulled out a sample expander from the cabinet. This bag was smaller than the implants and shaped more like an inflated disk. While I was coddling the bag, she continued her explanation.

"The size of the expander depends on the size of the breast you ultimately want—A, B, or C cup. This expander will have only a few ccs of saline inside when he first inserts it into your chest. We start small and expand the skin slowly."

I kept massaging the expander bag, trying to imagine this process.

"Every seven to fourteen days," she said, "you will come into the office, and Dr. F. will insert a needle into the expander and gradually add another few ccs, depending on how you're feeling."

This image made me flinch, but she had the discourse down pat. "The expander has a metal ring on the top. See here?" She pointed to a washer inlaid in the casing of the expander. "Inside this metal ring is a self-sealing piece of gauzelike fabric. When you come in for your injection of saline, Dr. F. will use a metal detector to find the metal ring. That way he'll know where to insert the needle."

When she paused for breath, I jumped in. "Let me get this straight. Dr. F. is going to use a stud finder to figure out where to inject the needle? Ingenious!" Of course, once again, a biomedical engineer of the male gender probably conceived the idea. I hated to admit what a clever idea it was.

"Do you know what size cup you want?"

"I'm thinking a B. I wear a C cup now, but I've had a lot of radiation and have been told my skin will not stretch very far."

"With a B, you'll need fewer injections. After each injection, it'll feel tight, but shouldn't hurt. When Dr. F. has injected enough saline in the expander, he'll wait at least two more weeks for the skin to loosen up a little bit more, and then we'll schedule the surgery."

I nodded, wondering how much time this would ultimately take.

"During this next surgery," she continued, "Dr. F. will replace the expanders with the implants and add on the nipple. He usually takes the skin for the nipple from your inner thigh. Then after the surgery, depending on the color of the transplanted skin, you can have the nipple tattooed to get a more realistic color contrast."

At this point, images of silicone bags, metal rings, needles, circular cutouts from my thigh, and tattoo needles in my nipple were swirling in my head. Somehow, all of this was going to add up to two perfect B-sized mounds with two realistically sculpted nipples. And this was the simple method?

The nurse responded to my bewildered gaze with a show of sympathy. "I know this sounds complicated, but Dr. F. has done this many, many times, and he's a master. You're in good hands. He'll talk with you shortly. Any questions so far?"

"No, not now. But I'm sure, as soon as I leave here, I'll think of a dozen."

"I'm always here to answer your questions. Call anytime. Each week, you'll see me first, so you can also bring your questions with you for the beginning of each visit."

And with that, she left the room. I liked her. She was helpful. She had delivered an easy-to-follow verbal guide to the Extreme Makeover for Breast-Be-Goners. She seemed sincerely interested in making this experience an informed and uncomplicated journey ending in optimal customer satisfaction. Now I was ready to meet the Master Sculptor.

Perched on the examining table in my clinic frock, I bided my time studying a child's drawing on the opposite wall. I was still staring at the drawing when Dr. F. walked in and introduced himself.

I asked, "Did your son do that drawing? He goes to University School with my daughter Shea, along with Jeanne Ballinger's son."

"Yes," he said with a huge father-proud grin. "He used to tell me, 'Steven's mommy takes the breasts off, and Daddy puts them back on!'"

The ice had been broken. We chuckled and dove into a discussion about the surgery. Dr. F. was quite animated about his work. Rodin could not have been more spirited about his artistic visions. Dr. F.'s explanations mirrored the nurse's, but with more graphic details about the cutting and pasting. He also mentioned the superior look of the silicone-filled implants, but again, there was no hard sell.

"I've got my mind made up," I said rather emphatically. "I want saline-filled implants."

That was that. He said no more about it.

"Dr. Ballinger told me you've had a lot of radiation." He gently kneaded the skin of my chest. "I don't think we'll have a problem, particularly with a size B. If you should decide you want the nipple colored, you will need to find a tattoo artist. Unfortunately, we don't perform the procedure here in the office."

"Where do I go?" I asked innocently.

"I don't really know. You'll need to ask the nurse about it. It can cost several hundred dollars, though, and insurance won't pay for it." (Years later some dauntless women led an effort resulting in a federal requirement for insurance providers to cover the tattoo cost.)

"It's up to you whether you want to get the nipple tattooed. I'll try and get a good sample of tissue with as much color contrast as possible. Let's look at your leg to see if we can take the skin graft for the nipple from the inside of your thigh."

I lay back on the examining table and pulled the gown open so he could see my inner thigh. His eyes landed on my oophorectomy scar that stretched across my lower belly about an inch above my pubic hair. He ran his forefinger over the scar.

"We can use the skin around this scar if you want, so we don't make another scar. You have quite a collection already!"

"This all sounds good to me—the implants, the nipple. After using a prosthesis for two years, I'm ready to go for it. No muss, no fuss—after you're done, that is."

I left the office feeling reassured, yet cautiously reserved. I was confident in my choice of sculpture and sculptor. Yet as I walked to my car, I felt a growing irritation with a word that had infiltrated my dialogue for the past several days. *Reconstruction.*

Reconstruction implied my beloved breasts could be restored. Can you reconstruct a stately old oak tree that has adorned your front lawn for decades? A mound sculpted from a fluid-filled bag and a numb piece of skin posing as a nipple doth not make a breast. It does make a mound, however.

Although I had an entire weekend to worry, the usual fear of the unknown preceding a major medical trauma was softened by my inflated sense of certainty in the outcome. I knew the cancer had been caught early. I knew the surgery would not be painful. I'd already experienced the loss of a bosom buddy. And I was weary of wrangling the burdensome detachable blob. I was ready to trade in the freedom of androgyny for a set of hassle-free mounds.

chapter eleven

1998, JANUARY

On January 18, 1998, the evening before my second mastectomy, Barry, Shea, and I checked into the Seton Inn at St. Thomas Hospital. The in-house hotel gave a welcome reprieve from a somber 4:30 a.m. drive into town on the morning of surgery. Instead, we had a leisurely dinner with Mom and Dad, followed by a tranquil evening. Barry, Shea and I snuggled into one of the two twin beds, hugging each other in a protective layer of silence marbled with love. After an hour or so, Shea crawled into the other bed, and a semi-serene slumber quickly befell us all.

The next day at 5:30 a.m., a nurse arrived to take me to the OR for Surgery Number Six. Barry and Shea got to sleep in. Now that's the way to start a surgical day.

I remember nothing about the surgery itself, which is a good sign. Unpleasant recollections are often all that remain of distant traumatic events. In the forty-eight hours after surgery, however, I recall a few unforgettable events. The first occurred when I awoke in a private hospital room. My entire body lay completely still except for my eyeballs. I looked to the left. I looked to the right. I looked to the end of my bed. I was alone.

I'm in a hospital room, I realized. *I'm in pain. I feel worse than shit. I feel awful.*

I turned my head toward the bed railing, and there she was, the gray cord leading to the control box with the magical button. I pressed the button labeled "nurse." And then I waited. And waited. In my overwhelming distress, it seemed like hours, but it might have been only a few minutes. I pushed the button again. No response. I started to moan. Moaning always diffuses discomfort. Then my fairy godfather Marshall, the anesthesiologist, dropped in from the clouds.

He stood over my bed and asked, "How you feeling, dear?"

"Not good," I whimpered. "I feel terrible. Achy all over. I feel like I'm going to pass out, even though I know I'm lying down."

"Sounds like your pain medicine has worn off. They need to get you on a pain pump. Have you called the nurse?"

"Yes. Twice. I don't think they even know I'm here."

"I'll be right back."

Marshall returned with the nurse.

"Let me check your chart. I'm pretty sure a pain pump has already been ordered for you," she said, then dashed out of the room. In my queasy state, I could feel her stress, and I was getting the sense the pace at St. Thomas Hospital had changed since my last superlative visit almost two years earlier.

Marshall held my hand. "They should not have let you lie here this long without giving you more pain medicine." His touch and his presence seemed to be intercepting the pain messages in my nerves.

"I feel better just knowing something is coming," I told him, "and that I'm not just left here to fend for myself. That was scary."

A few minutes came and went. Marshall left again to find help, and at length he came back with the harried, apologetic nurse.

In my previous visit to St. Thomas, I'd received attentive, compassionate, conscientious care, but now I caught glimpses of the New Age of Health Care—economized and downsized to an overworked, understaffed pool of providers. Over the next couple of days, I observed how a strong desire to serve gets watered down to numb mediocrity under severe stress—not a particularly good mission statement for a hospital: *to deliver mediocre care to as many people as we can as cheaply as we can.*

While the frazzled nurse hooked up the pain pump and tried to calmly explain how and when to use it, the urgent needs of her other patients seeped through her façade. Her tone was soft, but heavy with angst.

Within a couple of minutes, my sickly green state turned pink. Marshall squeezed my hand, gave me a kiss on my cheek, and left. Soon after, Barry and Shea were at my bedside. And then Mom and Dad. And then Ava. And then Kathleen. And then Rebecca. And then Jeanne. And then that was it for a while.

Apparently, I had cashed in most of the support equity with my friends and family during my first bout of breast cancer. The diehard devotees appeared at the end of my bed or sent flowers, but many who had made a personal visit in 1995 sent a card instead. My room felt emotionally bare with just two vases of flowers. I'm not complaining, just making an observation. After all, I wasn't as shaken by this event either.

Another vestige of Surgery Number Six was the tactile feel of the baggie stuffed *under* my stretched chest muscle and *on top of* my raw mastectomy wound. With the first mastectomy, the site of damage was left to heal naturally, unencumbered by foreign bodies. The discomfort after that surgery was almost nonexistent. This surgery, however, resulted in considerable pain. The contrast was striking. I could feel the shock of my wounded chest. She was rankled. *What in the heck are you doing to me? And you are doing this voluntarily? Tell me again, for what reason?*

There is a time and place for talking to your body parts. This was a befitting time. My wounded comrade deserved an explanation. I was trying to kill two mosquitoes with one swat. If I had waited for the left chest to heal before having the expander inserted, I'd be facing another surgery. Some upfront discomfort seemed like a small price to pay for avoiding one more date with the surgeon's knife. So I sent word, *Be patient, dear chest. This suffering now will result in a big return down the road.*

The last memento of this hospital stay was logged in on the morning of my third and final day. January 21, 1998, started out as one of those uneventful hospital days. Breakfast at 7:30 a.m., lovingly prepared with lukewarm scrambled eggs, soggy "wheat" toast, OJ diluted with melting ice, canal water coffee, and a carton of low-fat milk perfectly warmed to room temperature. I must confess, I love hospital food. Sans pain and discomfort, any food tastes heavenly in the sensory-deprived hospital milieu.

Hospital life can be sinfully luxurious, most notably the lack of a To Do list pressuring you to rally. The single, solitary goal is to lie in bed and heal. In this nurturing environment, one can eat and sleep and eat and sleep, as the body demands. This last lavish morning of my stay, I finished off the grub, pushed the hospital tray aside, and drifted off while still sitting up in bed. When I awoke, I was still alone. In a very relaxed state of mind, I leaned over, pressed the TV button, and turned my attention to the news.

As I listened to Dan Rather and the breaking story, I felt nauseated. He spoke of a woman whose name I had never heard. On the TV screen, Monica Lewinsky leaned over to hug President Clinton, standing out from the crowd in her black beret. As Mr. Rather filled us in on the meaning behind the innocent exchange, my heart sank with the emotional force of a distraught mother watching her firstborn strike out in a tie game of the Little League playoffs.

I was discharged later that morning, just as befuddled as the rest of America. After three nights and three days, the nurse instructed me how to siphon off the excess fluid draining through the tubes under both my arms. Then St. Thomas sent me home to heal, and also to watch the unfolding drama of Life in the Clinton White House. Even so, the call from Jeanne that all my nodes were negative for cancer alleviated my irritation toward the drain tubes *and* the Office of the President.

Reva, my faithful RN-sister-caretaker, came to town from Houston, relieving Barry from his duties as primary caregiver. Reva's visits always gave Barry the space he needed to navigate the postsurgical turmoil. This visit, however, tested the limits of Reva's tolerance. Upon her arrival, I was suffering from lethargic intestines, aka constipation. The pain meds had exacerbated the effects of the anesthesia, sedating the muscular walls of my intestines so they were unable to perform their gyrating dance to push the waste on down the line. Several sit-ins on the commode were the result.

Six days after discharge from the hospital, my intestines were still feeling sluggish, and I had settled in on the toilet with the *Bon Appetit* magazine in hand, hoping for success. As I strained to do the job, I felt a pop in my right ear—sort of like the pressure release you might hear when swooping down for the final descent in an airplane. Thus began Act I of what was to become the most challenging episode of my multi-decade medical journey.

A high-pitched, very low decibel ringing whirred in my ear after the pop. The tinnitus, as ringing in the ears is called, had an echo, as though a cup had been placed over my ear. Then suddenly, the end of my tongue went numb. The numbness gradually crept toward my cheek and spread out across the right side of my face. Still perched on the toilet, I lifted my arm to feel my face. What happened next came straight out of a creepy-crawling horror flick. My arm involuntarily began to flail about in circles. I watched my arm as if it belonged to someone—or something—else.

And then it hit me. *I'm having a stroke! Oh, this is really great.* I pleaded to myself and God, *Please, please, don't let me pass out. I don't want the paramedics making decisions without talking to me!*

My shoulders drooped toward my wounded chest with a cascading fatigue, while my buttocks settled farther into the toilet seat. I envisioned two paramedics squeezing into the tiny bathroom, trying to revive my limp, unconscious body lying on the white tile floor. I feared for my life, not only because of the possible stroke, but also because a less-than-adequate paramedic might inflict more damage.

I began to feel lightheaded, then dizzy. Just as I was about to pass out, my heavy, bobbing head dropped to my left shoulder. Without warning, the lightheadedness disappeared. But when I lifted my head, the dizziness returned. I quickly lowered my head to my shoulder again. The dizziness disappeared. *This is really odd.*

I yelled, "REEEVAAA!"

She was by my side in a jiffy.

"Uh. I don't feel so good. I feel like I'm going to pass out."

I began to fill her in on the details as I kept my head cocked to my shoulder. And then the nausea began to boil over.

She grabbed my hand. "Why don't you get off the toilet? Here, sit on the floor."

When I tried to move, up came the remains of Reva's homemade spinach lasagna I had devoured an hour earlier. I turned just in time to propel most of the recycled goodies into the toilet.

"Sorry, Reva. The lasagna was really good."

Then I threw up again.

Hanging over the toilet, I kept my head slightly cocked to the left, freeing Reva to clean up the splattered lasagna. As I write this, I still feel an aversion to spinach lasagna.

After the third round of vomiting, I slid to the floor, my head still hugging my shoulder. Then, reminiscent of my occasional migraines, an aura obscured the middle of my field of vision.

When I was able to catch my breath and tell Reva more, we both decided this evening's events were sponsored by one hellacious migraine. I sat on the floor for another half hour or so with Reva standing by. She called Jeanne, who concurred with the migraine theory for now, but she promised to call back after she talked with Seth.

Reva placed a warm, damp cloth on my forehead. I threw up one more time, and eventually the vomiting and dizziness stopped, and the numbness subsided. In their place was an excruciating headache on one side of my head, one of the worst migraines I had ever had. Two hours after I originally settled myself on the toilet with the *Bon Appetit*, Reva helped me to the bed and gave me some Phenergan and Percocet. I drifted into a deep sleep.

The ordeal ended just in time for Barry to take Reva to the airport to catch her plane back to Houston. I had done an outstanding job of making sure I got my money's worth out of her nursing services. When I awoke a few hours later, I felt like a new woman—a new woman who had been grabbed by the arms of Godzilla, swung round and round, mauled, then tossed heartlessly to the ground. Nonetheless, I felt better, with just a mild headache, fatigue, a little nausea, and numbness on the end of my tongue.

The next day brought no surprises. I laid low with a hangover. I avoided the bathroom. Danger lurked there. Jeanne called early that evening. She had talked with Seth, and they agreed a scan of the brain was the cautious thing to do, given my odd combination of neurological symptoms.

My first reaction, as usual, was a mixture of relief and its darker flipside, worry. Relief that I would not hover in the anxious unknown. Worry that I would soon lose the relief of ignorance. Attributing these events to a migraine was a stretch—a flailing arm, a numbed tongue and cheek, a loss of consciousness circumvented by a yogic meeting of my ear to my shoulder. These symptoms had never been in the repertoire of my twenty-five-year relationship with the migraine.

That same evening, Barry's parents, Chickie and Norm, drove in from Memphis to take the next shift as caregivers. We completed the round of welcome hugs and wasted no time loading up in the Corolla wagon to drive to St. Thomas Hospital for my brain scan. An MRI (magnetic resonance imaging) offered the most informative tour of the brain. There was concern, however, that the metal studs in my chest expanders might interfere with the magnetic charge of the MRI machine. The alternative, a CT scan (computerized axial tomography), used X-rays instead of magnetic fields, although the collective slices of images were not as revealing as the MRI.

By the time we arrived at the hospital, the long hallway from the lobby to the Imaging Clinic was dark, abandoned for the evening. All the clinic doors were closed. I passed no other patients or staff. Apparently I was the only lucky patient in need of the after-hours brain scan. The technician sitting at the reception area was ready and waiting for his customer.

After we introduced ourselves, he said, "I understand you recently had surgery for breast reconstruction. Is that correct?"

"Yes. I just had surgery ten days ago, and I had this weird seizure-like event last night." I was anxious to get some reaction, any reaction, to the significance of this event.

He revealed nothing. "Let's go ahead and get started. Have you ever had an MRI before?"

"No, I haven't. I've had beaucoup of other procedures, but somehow I have never needed an MRI, or any scan of the brain for that matter." I usually enjoyed launching into the most dramatic episodes of my medical saga at this point of introduction, but my mandibles were fatigued by the previous days' events.

I followed him into the next room. The MRI machine's long, cream-colored cylinder dominated the room. A narrow table extended from the machine's mouth, obviously where the body was positioned for transport through the tunnel. With its cramped three-foot diameter, the tunnel looked as inviting as a front-loading washing machine.

He patted the table with his hand. "Please lie down here."

I stretched out on the table as instructed. It amazed me that medical technicians could imagine comfort in the context of lying on a hard surface in a room frigid enough to keep meat from spoiling.

"What is an MRI exactly?" I asked.

The technician stood over me as he explained the procedure. "It's complicated, but it's mainly a set of three-dimensional images made by a powerful magnet transmitting radio waves through your tissues."

This explanation made some murky sense, but was not descriptive enough to help me visualize what was about to happen. The technician seemed oblivious to the shortfalls of his description as he focused on the work at hand. "I'm going to place these blocks around your head to hold your head in place. It's very important that you do not move your head. Even the tiniest movement may mean we'll need to do it over."

He placed a Naugahyde-covered block the size of a one pound bag of coffee on either side of my head. Then he placed a pillow under my knees and spread a blanket over my body. "It gets pretty cold in here. Will one blanket do it?"

"Thank you. I'm pretty cold. I sure would appreciate another blanket."

He grabbed another blanket and tucked me in. "Let me know if you need another one."

I thought, *So far, so good.*

He handed me a long cable with a button on the end. "Hold this in your hand so you can push the button if you need me. I'll be in the other room, but will stop the machine immediately if you push the button."

"Thank you."

"I'm going to put some earplugs in your ears. The machine makes a very loud clanging noise. Don't be scared. It's supposed to make that noise." He gently stuffed small, flesh-colored rubber earplugs in each of my ears, then said, "Here we go."

I could hear his muffled voice through the earplugs. He said, "I will slowly move you through the MRI machine and take one image at a time. It will probably take about thirty minutes to get all the way through."

I closed my eyes so I would not freak out from claustrophobia as he slid the table with my restrained head into the tunnel. He stopped just shy of my shoulders so that my head and neck were inside the tunnel, while the rest of my body was out on the limb. Although my eyes were closed, I could feel the entombment of the tunnel walls. I heard a door shut. I was alone. But then I heard his voice. "Are you okay?" he asked.

"Yes," I replied quickly, comforted by the proximity and clarity of his voice. Where was it coming from? It felt as though the machine was talking to me.

"Here we go. There will be a loud clanging."

The forewarning was just enough to keep me from leaping off the table—not that I could have since my head was trapped. I didn't even flinch. After two more outbursts from the machine, however, I felt as if an elephant was sitting on my chest about to pop my expanders. It was a baby elephant—not causing pain, just an intense, suffocating pressure.

I pushed the button, keeping my eyes sealed. The baby elephant got up. I heard the door open. I could feel the table and my body moving as he slid my head out of the tunnel. I opened my eyes. There was the technician, standing next to me.

"What happened?" he asked.

"I don't know. I felt this intense pressure on my chest."

"It may be the metal in the expanders." He looked truly puzzled about what to do next. "Do you want to try again?"

Do I **want** *to try again? Oh, yes. Let's do this again, because being trapped in a tunnel with Dumbo on my chest is an experience I* **want** *to do again.*

I kept my sarcasm to myself. "Yes," I whimpered. The procedure was necessary. Also, the power to shutdown the entire operation with just a push of a button gave me comfort.

So he adjusted the pillows next to my head and rolled me back into the tunnel. I closed my eyes and breathed deeply, intentionally. Breathe in. Hold. Release. Repeat. Breathe in. Hold. Release. My forefinger was on the button.

"Here we go," he warned.

Clang, clang, clang. Dumbo was back. I pressed the button.

He rolled me out. I opened my eyes and looked up at him. "I guess this is not going to work, huh?"

"No," he said. "We'll have to do a CT scan, which is right next door."

The experience of a CT scan is similar to an MRI but with a wider tunnel and without the clanging and banging. After about a half hour of slicing my brain into multiple three-dimensional images with the CT scan, he reappeared.

"I see a little something. Probably nothing, but I need to repeat the scan."

With his suspicious words, *I see a little something*, I lost the tangible link to the just-an-old-migraine scenario. In its place was raw fear. *I have brain cancer*, I thought. My fast conclusion was supported by the knowledge that breast cancer can metastasize to the brain. *My number has finally been called. My luck has run out. I'm burnt toast ready for the compost bucket. All right, Minda. Knock it off.*

Trying hard to hold back the tears, I squeaked, "You need to repeat it?"

"Yes," he said. "Have they ever picked up anything on a scan before?"

"No," I said nervously, then reminded him I'd never had a brain scan before.

"Well, let's repeat this scan. And then I'm going to inject a dye and do the scan again. It provides more contrast for better images. It's standard procedure."

Apparently, he had recognized his faux pas about revealing the "something suspicious" on the scan. We all have to learn from our mistakes. Fortunately, this new millennium has brought us experienced MRI and CT scan technicians who are more savvy about how and when to explain the purpose of a repeated scan. They also now know expanders and MRIs don't mix.

Ninety minutes later, I walked out of the Imaging Clinic. The technician said good-bye as he unsuccessfully tried to mask his concern. I cried the entire length of the dark hallway leading back to the waiting room, but before I emerged through the double doors to greet Barry, Chickie and Norm, I wiped my eyes and put on a poker face.

"All done," I said. Yet I couldn't hold back the news. "The technician said he saw something on the scan. I could tell by the look on his face that something is wrong."

"Oh, no, surely not. Let's think positive!" replied Chickie. She meant well, but her words held no credence. Barry and Norm looked worried, but said nothing. What was there to say?

"I'm starving. Let's go get a hamburger," I suggested. Red meat seemed like the best antidote.

Norm chose Wendy's, which was on the way home, and we decided to dine inside. The harsh fluorescent lights, too bright for a soothing ambience, burned the memory in place. A single quarter pounder, no cheese. I would have shoved the entire square patty and round bun in my mouth at once if I could have, it tasted so good. Hamburger is comfort food, a concept I fully embraced on that cold January evening.

In the car on the way home, I called our friend Becca from Barry's new-fangled cell phone, his first. We hoped Becca, who was Seth's nurse practitioner, could help us connect the dots. She suggested I call Tom John, a mutual friend and St. Thomas physician who could access the radiologist's report by phone. Tom jumped on the mission and called back in a few minutes to let us know the report wasn't back yet. The phone rang again a looooong five minutes later.

"I got the radiologist's report," Tom said. "It looks like a tumor called an acoustic neuroma. This is not necessarily bad news. This type of tumor is almost always benign."

A cold, overcast day can set the stage for the doldrums. Or the same cold, cloudy day can be a glorious time to be alive. In a common coping mechanism, I came back home with the latter perspective, physically exhausted, but mentally ecstatic. I had not had a stroke. My breast cancer was gone. And cancer was *not* encroaching on my brain.

Barry and his parents were relieved also. All of us were oblivious to the ramifications of a tumor lodged between my brain stem which controls the heart and lungs, and the numerous cranial nerves controlling my hearing, tasting, tearing, balance, and facial movement. Ignorance was the best medicine. In retrospect, I am very thankful I was kept in the dark about the full ramifications of this not-so-innocent, benign tumor until long after my chest had healed.

We headed home, and I went straight to the bathroom where I had the biggest dump I had had since before the surgery. With the passage of several days of food waste, I released all of the tension of the previous thirty hours. One minute I had been convinced the cancer demons were back. The next minute I was given yet another reprieve. I felt vague but unwavering faith that I still had a few lives left.

On Monday, I consulted with Dr. B., a neurologist and another fine example of a physician who approached her livelihood with sincere compassion and engaging dialogue. Her explicit explanations instilled confidence in her recommendations. We talked for at least an hour.

"There are several possible scenarios for what happened last week," she said. "The important thing now is to get to the bottom of it so we can protect you from any conditions that could have more catastrophic results down the road."

She handily laid out all the pieces of this complex puzzle, transforming several story lines into a tight script. She didn't frighten me or leave me wanting more information. Stroke, hematologic disorder, embolism, neurofibromatosis, acoustic neuroma, Valsalva maneuver. None of these labels set off the panic button. Her logical explanations and recommendations for follow-up comforted my vulnerable psyche.

The next steps for solving the puzzle boiled down to two referrals. First, Dr. C., a cardiologist, was to perform a trans-esophageal echocardiogram and take blood samples to check for evidence of a clotting disorder or embolism (obstruction) in my heart that may have caused my "stroke in a young person." The second referral to Dr. Gary Jackson, a surgeon specializing in the skull base, would determine whether the tumor in my head was, in fact, an acoustic neuroma. This type of tumor was generally slow growing and secondary in concern to a possible cardiac problem.

I scheduled the appointment with the cardiologist for a few weeks away. It had been two weeks since the mastectomy, and I was ready to return to My Year Off, shunting everything physical out of my mind. Enough of this drama. I was no longer gainfully employed beyond teaching one nutrition class at Vanderbilt. But my year's plan of a lightened load, serving as director of Shea's May Bat Mitzvah weekend and my own respite, had been mightily invaded by the breast cancer, reconstruction, and yet-to-be-named brain tumor.

My schedule became rather erratic. One day I was the devoted chauffeur and mentor, escorting Shea to Hebrew lessons, her Warner Park community service project, or the eternal search for "the dress" for her Bat Mitzvah party. The next day I was giving a lecture to Vandy nursing students on prenatal and infant nutrition. The day after that, I was gliding in and out of Shea's volleyball and softball games, slumber parties, and Mother-Daughter Book Club meetings. Another day, I'd be at yoga class, my feet and arms planted firmly on the floor a shoulder's width apart as I assumed my wimpish version of downward-facing dog—all my body could handle.

Sprinkled throughout this irregular schedule was an odd assembly of corporeal happenings. Every two weeks, I lay on the examining table as Dr. F. rubbed the stud finder across my mounds to find the metal opening. He then injected saline, slowly expanding the temporary mounds and skin. Each time, I left the office with a chest as full as a breastfeeding mama who had not seen her baby since yesterday.

My skin felt as if a tourniquet had been tied around my chest, and I was afraid to inhale too deeply for fear of bursting the bags. Relief from the achy stretching came within twenty-four hours, though, as the skin extended enough to ease the tension.

One time per month, I made a visit to Marty, a healing touch practitioner. The touch, which was clearly healing, began with a series of movements of Marty's hands a few inches over and on my body as I lay face up on a massage table. After a baseline assessment of the flow of energy through my seven energy centers, or chakras, she passed her hands over my body to help clear the "field," open the chakras, and balance the energy flow.

Though skeptical at first, I became a believer after the first treatment. It felt as though she had reached into my chest and lifted out several handfuls of gunk. A clean, airy lightness replaced the dense jam she seemed to have dislodged. By the end of the treatment, I left her house with a bounce in my step, as if awakened from a refreshing afternoon siesta. Although subsequent treatments were not as dramatic as the first, there was a consistent aftereffect. I always felt rested and renewed, with a velvety movement of breath through my body.

In between mound expansion and the healing touch, the acoustic neuroma began to plead for attention in several peculiar ways. My left eyelid that had twitched on and off for a couple of years was gaining speed and fluttering nonstop for hours at a time. Then a new sensation surfaced. An imaginary pool of saliva settled into one corner of my lips.

I could not get the image out of my head of the boy who sat behind me in Miss Dunavant's fourth grade class at Richland Elementary. He always grossed me out with the white bubbly fluid forever wedged in the corners of his ridiculous smirk. In truth, there was no saliva resting in my smile. The tumor was just pressing on one of my cranial nerves controlling the feeling to my lips and cheek, causing a tingling sensation.

The unnamed mass also poked its elbows into my balance nerve so that I began to feel a little tipsy in the dark. Occasionally, I tripped on phantom steps, and walls suddenly appeared before my face as I turned corners. One day, while combing the aisles of Jo Ann's Fabrics for Bat Mitzvah decorations, I had to drop to the floor to keep from passing out. The lightheadedness usually presented itself when I was out and about, such as in the midst of rows of ribbons and fabric paints.

With these frequent reminders, Ms. Brain Tumor was squeezing herself into my personal peace of mind. I got serious about a daily practice of meditation and mental imagery to give myself some feeling of control. Each morning I sat in the familiar cross-legged pose on the blue zafu cushion atop the pale yellow Chinese rug in our bedroom. My mind's eye followed a few consciously deep breaths moving into my nostrils and down my trachea, expanding my lungs and filling the cul-de-sacs of my bronchioles. I shifted into reverse as the breath moved out, carrying away the particles of debris from the angst of the previous twenty-four hours. Pranayama, or intentional breathing, is a conscious attempt to submerge oneself in a daily bath of pure, warm, oxygen-laden breath that spreads throughout the body until every drop of dirty, unwanted matter has twirled into oblivion. Breathing in and out is the easiest imagery of all.

After a few breaths cleared the way, I envisioned bright orange-red lava seeping from the top of my head down into the right side. Without clarity about the exact location of the tumor, I let the hot, healing lava flood the area around my middle and inner ear.

The need to coddle my body did not let up. My brain CT scan had revealed three lesions in my cerebellum, indicating I had experienced three small strokes sometime in my past. The combination of these lesions and the neurological symptoms during the bathroom caper worried Dr. B. Was I at risk for another stroke? So in the spring of 1998, my heart went on display via a transesophageal echocardiogram to search for a possible blood clot or "vegetation" poised and ready to trigger another stroke.

The purpose of the transesophageal echocardiogram was to get a better look at the heart from the *inside* of my chest as opposed to an echocardiogram from the *outside*. Just prior to the visit to the cardiologist, when I finally grasped the full intent of the referral, my rationalizing became quite imaginative. As can happen when one is freaked out and under-informed, I put three and three together and made ninety-nine. I heard the word *vegetation* and assumed they were looking for a growth that would require open heart surgery. No one had mentioned open heart surgery, yet the threat loomed as real as the tumor in my head. As I was given the hospital gown, I was so nervous, I asked for Valium.

"That's an unusual request for this procedure," said the nurse, "but I'll check with the doctor."

He obliged. The Valium relieved my strained mind and relaxed my taut muscles. After sedation of brain and body, the procedure was over within thirty minutes. My heart was pumping like a forty-year-old, the cardiologist said. No heart surgery was in my near future. Despite the recent breast cancer and current brain tumor, I was thrilled with this new lease on life. Later, in researching the medical records for this book, I was a bit deflated when I read the cardiologist's notes stating she *looks her age of 42* with a *mildly aesthetic habitus*. I beg your pardon, Dr. C., my husband tells me my habitus is pretty awesome!

The following week, I attended a support group meeting of breast cancer survivors, sponsored by the local chapter of the American Cancer Society. As these women took turns telling their stories, I felt as unsympathetic as a homeless Katrina victim listening to the accounts of rain showers. My dearth of compassion gave me qualms, but to me, their stories of trauma sounded like whining. Most of them were not in imminent danger of dying. Of course they had valid reasons to whine, but I thought I had valid reasons not to care. Regrettably, I left the group feeling estranged from my breast cancer sisters.

A few weeks later, Barry and I went in for my first visit with Dr. Gary Jackson, the physician whose nimble hands would affect my well-being almost as much as all of the other doctors combined thus far. A neurotologic skull base surgeon, he was one of the most experienced acoustic neuroma surgeons in the country.

Dr. Jackson was a large man with a large presence. He walked into the small clinic room, introduced himself, and sat down on the padded stool. He confirmed that my2.2-centimeter tumor was an acoustic neuroma of the midsize variety, operable with microsurgery. That sounded innocuous. He said the surgery could be delayed until after my breast reconstruction was complete. He added that, in general, this surgery was not complicated. Barry and I walked out with the impression this new nugget would be no big deal.

We were so saturated with medical details from the breast cancer, reconstruction, and possible stroke that we failed to comprehend removal of this tumor would require cutting through my skull. In retrospect, I realize Dr. Jackson was sparing us stress by not revealing the magnitude of this surgery. He wisely realized our cup had runneth over. In a letter he wrote to Dr. B., the referring neurologist, he captured the situation:

> In all honesty, like you, I probably don't know what her life expectancy is, but I expect it to be long enough to be concerned about the size of the acoustic. This woman and her family have been through hell and back and are trying to come to a reasonable decision.

Dr. Jackson would later become my knight in shining armor. For the next few months, however, I tucked visions of my acoustic neuroma and coming surgery in an unreachable corner of my mind. Caterers, printers, and table decorations were beckoning as Shea's Bat Mitzvah ceremony approached.

chapter twelve

1998, MAY

On May 23, 1998, our shy, precious thirteen-year-old miracle child stood up before the synagogue congregants, family, and friends and was inducted into the not-so-exclusive club of bona fide Bat Mitzvahs. In the southern traditions of this Jewish rite of passage, becoming a Bat (or Bar) Mitzvah is a unique amalgamation of spiritual awakening, community service, initiation into adulthood, family reunion, and materialistic decadence. As reasonably grounded, mildly observant Reform Jews, we chose the middle ground for a meaningful, festive celebration.

Friends and family from Atlanta to LA joined the Micah congregation as Shea took to the pulpit. With the poise of a seasoned scholar, she led the congregation through the service, reading her Torah and singing her Haftorah portions, and articulating her thoughts on the meaning of the ritual. When it was time for the parental sermon from the ark, I stood before Shea and shared some wise words I thought might possibly penetrate a preteen's ears.

"Shea, when I stopped to think about why I thought it was important for you to become a Bat

Mitzvah, many things came to mind. Most important, I want you to have the same advantages I had growing up in the Jewish faith. I've not told you this before (don't worry, I'm not going to embarrass you), but when I was in high school and was diagnosed with cancer, I was scared. You know how the sight of blood gives you the heebie-jeebies? Well, when I was a teenager with cancer, I got the heebie-jeebies, too. So when I got scared, I would just close my eyes and say the Sh'ma."

I closed my eyes and began chanting the first couple of lines of the prayer, "Sh'ma Yisrael Adonai Eloheinu Adonai echad . . ." I opened my eyes and locked gazes with Shea again.

"When I chanted the Sh'ma, suddenly I would feel better, stronger. I would feel a connection to something bigger than myself, a strong connection to my family, to hundreds of years of tradition. It would give me so much strength. Pretty powerful stuff. I want you to have that, too, when you need it . . ."

I stepped back from the pulpit to my appointed seat on the Bema, quite proud of myself—mission accomplished! I hoped that I had inspired Shea one small step farther into a spiritual awakening. Years later when I asked her what she remembered most about her Bat Mitzvah service, she replied, "When it was over . . . the rabbi's speech . . . and your eyelid twitching the whole time you were talking to me." She didn't remember the content of my speech because my twitching eyelid distracted her. Oh, well.

Ironically, I was distracted, too. Not by my fluttering eyelid, but by the greatly inflated mounds in my chest. I was reaching the end of the expander injections, so my chest was resting so high it seemed almost to reach my chin. My new big mamas reminded me of our Eastern European grandmothers. Generous bosoms were the first things you noticed when these elder women hugged you. In my case, the overinflated mounds were so hard and unyielding, I felt like a bouncing ball each time I embraced one of our guests. At each impact, my body recoiled backward — Boing!

A few days after the Bat Mitzvah, I was ready to turn my attention back to my body. I had not yet grasped the scale of the physical challenges that lay ahead with the brain tumor surgery, so my Type-A personality was driving me to bring the mound construction and acoustic neuroma projects to a close.

I had two more visits with the breast sculptor, Dr. F., to squeeze in a few more vials of saline. By the end of June, my skin was stretched as tightly as the pigskin of a football. The goal was to create a pocket on each side of the chest to accommodate the B-sized implants with a little extra room for comfort. After the final injection, Dr. F. gave my chest six weeks off before the big switcharoo to the permanent saline implants.

"Now, you can rest and relax," he said as he squeezed the final saline into my chest. "Let's give your skin a chance to respond to the stretching."

On this last visit before the surgery, we took a closer look at the options for skin transplants to sculpt the nipples, and I consented to using spare tissue through the existing scar at the bottom of my tummy, the only external evidence of the abduction of my ovaries.

Dr. F. passionately explained his craft in more detail by outlining each of the steps for constructing a fake breast complete with a nipple-like protrusion in the center.

Step 1.	Reopen the left side of the chest at the site of the mastectomy scar.
Step 2.	Lift out the saline-filled temporary expander from beneath the pectoral muscle.
Step 3.	Insert the permanent B-sized saline-filled implant, and wiggle it into place.
Step 4.	Sew up the opening, leaving a gap in the center for the insertion of the "nipple."
Steps 5-8.	Repeat steps 1 through 4 on the right side.
Step 9.	Reopen the belly just above the pubic hairs at the site of the existing scar.
Step 10.	Cut out two circles of skin about one and one half inches in diameter.
Step 11:	Reseal the belly.
Step 12.	Stitch a circle into one of the circular skin transplants with self-dissolving thread about one-third of an inch from the center. Then gently pull on the stitch to gather the circle like a tiny purse, resembling a nipple-like protrusion. Tie a knot to hold the "nipple" in place.
Step 13.	Sew the circle into the center of the new mound on the left side.
Steps 14-15.	Repeat steps 12 and 13 on the right side.

On the morning of August 8, 1998, I checked into the Baptist Hospital Women's Center for the final fifteen-step "reconstruction" of the mounds. In two hours, I would be a new and improved version of my former self! Demolishing the old to make way for the new—this two-year journey of urban renewal for the chest was about to come to a close.

The Women's Center felt more like a clinic than a hospital. When Barry and I walked in, he sat down in the lobby while I checked in with the receptionist. Mound factories were efficient. Within a few minutes, we were called back into an examining room. The attendant gave me a hospital gown, instructing me to take off everything and put on the gown with the opening in the front.

"I'll be back in a few minutes to talk with you about the surgery and get your signature on the release forms." Sure enough, she came back in a few minutes.

"Dr. F. will be in shortly. He is *so* good at this. You're in great hands. He'll do a few measurements to help assure the breasts and nipples are centered, and then off you'll go to the operating room. The surgery will take around ninety minutes. After the surgery, you'll be taken to a room in the hospital, and if all goes well, you will go home tomorrow. Any questions?"

"No questions. I'm ready to get the show on the road!"

She pointed to the obligatory "it is not our fault" papers in the event of an unforeseen detour. "If you'll sign here and here, and initial here, here, here, here, and here, you'll be on your way."

I signed the papers. Out she went, and in came Dr. F. with the Jerry Lewis smirk that surgeons often wear in the final meet-and-greet prior to the showdown.

"Good morning! How are you feeling today?"

I sat on the edge of the examining table, and he pulled up a stool next to me.

"I'm great. Ready to get this over with."

He slid his stool just inches away from my chest so his eyes aligned with my about-to-burst mounds protruding from the gown. "Let me have a look at your chest. I'm going to draw on your chest to mark where I'll place the nipples."

As he turned to the table with his tools, I opened the gown to give him a full frontal view. He grabbed a black plastic bottle cap from the tray (he was a plastic surgeon, after all) and fixed his eyes on my left mound for what seemed like an eternity. Master Sculptor Monsieur Rodin was envisioning where to place his chisel. Then he placed the bottle cap on the center of my left mound and traced a circle around the bottle cap with a fine-tip Sharpie.

"We're talking high-tech here," I said, rather shocked.

"They actually make an expensive kit with templates and marker, but I've found plastic bottle caps work just fine." A frugal, resourceful perfectionist—not what I expected from a plastic surgeon—but I was pleased with his craftiness. He glared a minute at the other mound and then drew the second circle.

I suddenly got worried as I looked down at my chest and saw the cockeyed circles. "They're not even!"

"Don't worry," he replied in a self-assured manner. "Remember, we've stretched out the skin as far as it will go, but each side has not responded exactly the same. Notice that the right side looks a bit higher than the left. So I have to estimate where the center will be *after* the expanders have been replaced with the implants and the swelling goes down. I'm actually pretty good at hitting the target," he said proudly.

In this case, pride was good. I did not want to hear, *Sometimes I'm a good marksman, and sometimes I'm not.*

"Wow," I said, "this is quite an art." I had not given a thought until that moment about how he was going to assure the nipples ended up in the right place.

"Okay. We're ready to go," he said as the nurse brought in the gurney. "Let's get you over to the operating room. Any other questions?"

"No. I don't think so." I started to feel excited about the birth of my nippled twin mounds.

As he and the nurse were rolling me out the door, he pointed to my belly and asked, "Would you like for me to do a little liposuction on some of the fat around the scar? While I have you open, it's easy to do."

"Go for it!" I exclaimed. *What a deal!* I was all smiles as they rolled me away to the OR. His special one-time offer was the last thing I remember before I woke up in the hospital bed.

"Oooooooooooh," I moaned to whoever would listen. I could not see my chest, but I could feel her. She was a wounded animal who had been stomped by a predator. I felt no sharp pains, just a solid mass of achiness that extended from my neck to my solar plexus. I turned to see who was next to me, and there was my beloved nuclear family—Barry, Mom, and Dad. Shea was in school.

I drifted off. I woke up a couple of hours later and regrounded myself in the new hospital room. I asked Barry, "Would you open my gown? I'd like to see my chest."

Barry helped me pull the gown open. My chest was wrapped in an eight-inch swath of gauze. For now, I could only imagine the Monsieur's masterpieces hidden beneath the layers of cotton.

When the nurse came in, I asked, "When will I be able to see them?" I still could not bring myself to call them breasts. My breasts were long gone. These mounds were impostors. Much wanted and welcomed impostors, but not the real things.

She said, "Not until your first office visit when the bandages are changed."

The next day I felt pretty sore, but ready to go home. Once again I received instructions before I was discharged for stripping and draining the four tubes.

Over the next few months, and now years, I gradually got to know and appreciate my new buddies. Like any new friends, once the honeymoon is over, both the good and the bad settle out. Hopefully, the good outweighs the bad. This was the case for me and my mounds.

The Good:

1.   Saline-filled baggies defy gravity. Although the mounds did not have the relaxed, shapely physique and softness of their

predecessors, they filled up my blouse in a most attractive way.

2.   Dr. F. was a damn good craftsman. It took many months for the swelling to settle and the mounds to find their center of gravity, but when they did, the faux nipples were perfectly centered.

3.   A boon no one forewarned me about still amazes me as I write this. My perky little babies required no support. I stuffed all of my bras in the back of the drawer. Free at last!

The Bad:

1.   Saline-filled baggies defy gravity. The same feature that turned me into a braless freedom rider also resulted in mounds that assumed the same stance year after year after year. My baggies looked like the same tennis balls in the new millennium as they did at their birth in 1998. I was hoping for a little droop to give them a more natural look. That feature usually comes with the silicone model, a choice I had scorned. I made an informed choice for valid reasons, so I have accepted the less than perfect mounds.

2.   Medical insurance did not cover the cost of the tattoo artist. One of my fake nipples eventually assumed one shade darker than the surrounding skin. The other one did not. An expensive dye-job for my faux

areolas was not a high priority. I was fiscally and physically wasted after the triad of surgeries, so it was difficult to summon the oomph to take this step.

The Ugly:

1.   The nurse handed me a policy describing the lifetime guarantee. The baggies were guaranteed for life from leakage, but, as with most policies, one must read the fine print. With the generous prior record of the implant manufacturers, it should come as no surprise the guarantee covered the baggie, but not the surgery to replace the baggie!

Mentor H/S will replace its all-saline-filled mammary implants due to deflation or due to loss of shell or valve integrity during the lifetime of the patient-recipient upon request. . . This replacement policy is limited to replacement of the Mentor H/S all-saline-filled mammary prosthesis and Mentor H/S shall not be responsible for any incidental or consequential damages of any kind, directly or indirectly, arising from the use of this product, including without limitation, medical, surgical and hospital costs. . . .

~ Lifetime Replacement Policy,
Mentor H/S, Santa Barbara, CA, April 1996

3.   The manufacturers of the baggies had not
        worked out the wrinkles. Within a year
        after my surgery, the baggie deflated on the
        left side of my right breast, forming a small
        ditch the size of a short, thin pencil. No
        sweat. It certainly was not worth another
        surgery to have the baggie replaced,
        particularly if I had to pay the surgeon, the
        hospital, and the anesthesiologist to retrieve
        and replace the goods.

4.   The skin transplant relocated from my
        lower abdomen to the center of the right
        mound came with a bonus—a pubic hair.
        About once a month, I plucked the loner.
        But it always grew back.

When all was said and done, I was a satisfied
customer. The advantages far outweighed the
disadvantages. When I got dressed in the morning, I
buttoned up my blouse, *always* pleased with the
decorative bulges. Toward summer's end when the
construction project was complete, the saga of my
radiated breasts was history. They were gone. I moved
on. I turned my attention to the tumor lodged in my
head.

I was entering year twenty-eight of my medical
soap opera. These many years of experience, wisdom
and confusion rolled into one lumpy ball, and the older
I got, the more frequently I was forced to sort out
ordinary signs of aging from obscure warnings of
catastrophic disease.

Lightheadedness, loss of balance, a twitching eyelid, and a phantom pool of saliva perched on my lip, these symptoms rotated in and out for months. It had been easy to blow aside these curious little markers of neurological upheaval while I was finding my way through Breast Cancer Number Two—until the bathroom caper forced me out of denial. The effect was short-lived, though. I picked myself up and walked right back to the safe side of denial, allowing my battle-fatigued psyche a respite. Yes, a tumor was pressing on my brain stem, but I did not, could not, and would not acknowledge what was required to get it out. Yet once the Bat Mitzvah, breast cancer, and mound construction were behind me, it was time face the next demon.

chapter thirteen

1998, AUGUST

In August of 1998, I began a tumultuous three-year journey that mangled my body and jarred my soul. By this point, I was worn out, trying to hold on, but almost ready to let go. I flippantly warned Barry again and again, "If one more physical assault comes my way, I'm out of here!" I felt no sadness about the potential loss of life. In fact, much of the time, I felt blissful. One more day or four more decades—it didn't seem to make a difference.

Thirteen days following the surgery for the mound construction, I finally began my journey in earnest toward ousting the latest mass of unwanted cells. I had a repeat of the MRI attempted earlier, followed by balance and hearing tests and a consultation with Dr. Jackson, the surgeon.

Seven months had passed since the initial diagnosis. Barry and I were forced to acknowledge Dr. Jackson would have to reach inside my skull to pluck out the tumor. We felt like such idiots that we had not grasped this concept sooner. We did not let on to Dr. Jackson how shocked we really were when he described the procedure of drilling a hole through my skull. He had mentioned *microsurgery* before. Microsurgery sounded small. Simple. We'd assumed he would go through the ear canal and pluck it out. How difficult could something requiring tiny surgical tools be? We never sought an answer to that question until we sat with Dr. Jackson on that August day.

"You have three choices," he said, "surgically remove the tumor through a microsurgical approach, shrink it with radiation, or leave it there and just watch it."

Barry and I exchanged glances.

"Given your age and the size of the tumor, I do not recommend the latter," Dr. Jackson said. "It will only become more difficult to remove as it gets larger. Also, given the amount of radiation you've already received to the neck, I suspect radiation is not an option either, although you may want to check that out further."

I nodded, though I felt pretty sure radiation was out.

The doctor continued, "From a surgical standpoint, if a tumor has been radiated and grows back, it becomes very difficult to go back in and remove the tumor surgically."

"Is there a difference in the recurrence rate of radiated tumors versus surgically removed ones?" I asked, trying hard to focus on one issue while the various scenarios were chaotically colliding in my brain.

"Yes. The rate is lower among the surgically removed tumors, although they haven't been using radiation on acoustic neuromas long enough to get a good handle on the true risk of a recurrence."

He pointed to a chart on the wall which contained a graphic rendering of the inside of the skull from the outer ear to the brain stem. A lot was happening in that tiny span, so he gave us a little orientation. Here's what we learned.

The external ear is connected to the ear canal, which is connected to the eardrum, which is connected to the middle ear (ear bones), which is connected to the inner ear (labyrinth). Then, running through a gap between the inner ear and the brain stem is the acoustic nerve, whose job is to assure a smooth transfer of sound data to the brain. This nerve also controls balance.

In Mother Nature's efficient fashion, several other nerves are squeezed into this space. These cranial nerves, as they are called, carry messages from the head and neck to the brain and sometimes back out again. All are numbered (by us, not Mother Nature), and the ones snuggling up most closely to nerve VIII, the acoustic nerve, are nerves VI, VII, IX, and X. They control eye movement, sensation of the mouth and face, production of tears and saliva, movement of the facial muscles, taste sensation, and swallowing.

With all this inherently important activity displayed before me, I stood up and asked, "Where exactly is this tumor? I know you've described this to me before, but I'm still confused."

He pointed to the acoustic nerve. "This nerve branches into two parts, as you can see here. One part controls your hearing, and the other part controls your balance. Your tumor has grown here, from the end of your inner ear to your brain stem."

He then swiveled his stool toward the desk and grabbed a flesh-colored, fist-size model of the brain. He pointed to the brain stem, the third chamber of the brain extending down from the cerebellum. "Your tumor is now actually pressing on your brain stem, causing it to bend, like this." He made a C with his thumb and forefinger. "It's causing moderate pressure on the brain stem. It's not a small and not a large tumor, 2.2 centimeters—which we call a medium-size tumor."

Large, medium, small, the Three Bears came to mind. My tumor was Mama Bear, and the difficulty of getting to it was coming into focus.

I said, "If we leave it alone, will it possibly go away?" I was hoping for a simple yes, so I could scratch the impending surgery off my To Do list.

"I've never seen that happen," he replied. "Acoustic neuromas usually are very slow-growing tumors. They can remain dormant for a while, which is why some people choose not to remove them. Unfortunately, they can have a growth spurt at any time. In your case, the pressure on the brain stem suggests to me it should be removed."

When he saw the look on my face, he explained that the brainstem controlled the crucial functions of heart rate and respiration. "The greater the pressure on the brain stem," he said, "the more serious the potential problems can be. If you were many years older, you might consider the wait-and-see route. But at forty-three, you're young, and I hope you have a long life ahead."

"Hm," I said, stalling for time, hoping a reasonably intelligent question would spin my mind away from the unfolding anarchy. "You've talked about microsurgery. How does that work?"

"With microsurgery, there are two points of entry into the skull," he said. "Each has its advantages and disadvantages. In your case, I would suggest the translabyrinth approach where we go in behind your ear through the mastoid bone."

He pointed once again to the drawing. "The translab approach is the most direct way, and it allows us to see the tumor most clearly. But we have to remove the middle and inner ear structures. So it will cause deafness in that ear."

He paused and waited for a reaction. I was silent, baffled not only by the news of the deafness, but also by the complexity of the surgery. Barry seemed even more jarred. As a musician, he was horrified by the possibility of total hearing loss in one ear.

Barry probed, "Is hearing loss an absolute or just a possible outcome?"

"With the translab approach, we take out the hearing nerve, so hearing will not be preserved on that side." Then Dr. Jackson turned toward me. "If you were a singer or musician, I would probably suggest consideration of a newer approach through the middle fossa that might give you a pretty good chance of preserving your hearing."

He pointed to a spot farther above the ear. "With this method, the ear structures are left intact, and the brain is elevated to expose the tumor. But in your case, given the size and location of your tumor, I think the translab approach would be best."

NO COMPLICATIONS was flashing in big red neon lights. This was a no-brainer for me—good thing because information from my brain was flowing slower than catsup from a newly opened bottle.

"Well," I said, "I'm most concerned about getting it all out and making sure there are as few complications as possible. Hearing loss is not a problem for me if it gives you the best shot for doing this. I'll still be able to hear out of the other ear."

Despite the size of the tumor, I had not yet experienced noticeable loss of hearing, so I was ignorant of the full impact of one-ear deafness.

I continued, "The approach you recommend makes sense. I'd like to get a second opinion, though. I hope you know, a second opinion doesn't reflect a lack of confidence in your surgical abilities. I just know from previous experience I want to walk into this surgery as confident as possible that I've chosen the right man and the right procedure for the task."

"If you want a second opinion, you ought to go to the best." Then he told us about the House Ear Clinic in LA, named for Dr. Howard P. House who did much of the pioneering work on surgical techniques for removal of acoustic neuromas. His protégé, Dr. B., probably performed more acoustic neuroma surgeries than anyone else in the world. "I'll get you his number," Dr. Jackson said.

"What are the side effects of the trans . . . what did you call it?"

"Translabyrinth—we cut across the labyrinth of the inner ear."

"So what are the side effects, other than loss of hearing?"

"There could be damage to other nerves. Regardless of how we enter the skull, there will be some tugging, fraying, or cutting of the neighboring nerves. The cranial nerves are very tiny and are right next to each other. How well I am able to separate the tumor from the other nerves largely depends on the tumor itself—whether it's a good guy or a bad guy. The good guys lift out with minimal damage. But if I have to extract it in pieces, there will probably be more damage to the other nerves, particularly the facial nerve."

"What would that mean?" I asked.

"Damage to this nerve causes facial weakness, and in the worst cases—if the tumor's wrapped around the facial nerve, for instance—there may be total facial paralysis. Hopefully, any damage will be temporary."

Yes, hopefully, I thought.

He said, "When we get inside, we'll place a monitor on these other nerves that buzzes when I disturb them. This monitor helps me minimize the damage. In the unlikely event I have to cut the entire facial nerve to remove the tumor, we can do some repair by grafting a portion of another nerve. This happens only in a very small percentage of cases."

So far, he had not said anything that shook me up enough to reroute my brain to la-la land. Naïvely, temporary loss of my face muscles did not sound too traumatic, so I innocently moved on to probe for the worst. "Are there other side effects?"

"There's a small chance of a blood clot forming and causing a stroke, particularly since your tumor is pressing on the brain stem. It rarely happens—less than one percent of the time."

Gulp.

"The translab approach keeps that risk to a minimum," he added, observing the concern my fully functioning facial muscles conveyed.

I studied the scribbles on the sheet of paper I had brought with me. I did not want to make eye contact. I felt he had exposed some deep, dark secret that embarrassed us both. For serious medical risks, even one percent is worrisome. I looked over my list of questions, waiting for the awkwardness of the uncomfortable news to pass. I asked for the worst, but was hoping for nothing. I waited a moment longer until I regained my composure, reviewing my list again and again.

"I've been doing research on choosing surgeons," I said, "so I hope you'll be patient with me as I go through my list here."

"No problem, Mrs. Lazarov. I'm here to help you understand as much as possible about your choices and your ultimate decision."

"How many of these surgeries do *you* actually do, not just assist with or supervise?"

"I remove one to two acoustic neuromas a week. These surgeries take all day, some six to seven hours, some many more."

"How long do you think mine will take?"

"I can only guess at this point as I need to look more closely at the MRI. But I'm guessing eight or nine hours. The first part alone to get inside the skull will take at least four hours. Then we have to remove the mastoid bone and clear the rest of the way to the tumor. How long it takes to remove the tumor depends on whether it's a good guy or a bad guy. Then we cut a piece of fat from another part of your body to help plug the hole in the skull and close everything up."

At this point I was thinking, *Too bad I didn't save a sample from my recent liposuction.*

"The surgery will actually be on the video monitor in the waiting room," he said, "so your family can watch if they want."

"Wow. Thank you, Dr. Jackson. We've got much to think about. I think you are my man, but I would like to talk with Dr. B."

"Let's walk out to the nurses' desk, and I'll ask them to get his number for you." He stood up, then we stood up—in proper order, like courtiers in waiting for the king.

I actually felt pretty good. I liked Dr. Jackson. He played it straight, answering my questions in terms I could understand, without sugarcoating the answers. He also did not make me feel uncomfortable for probing. I could tell he took his work very seriously, with pride and confidence in his abilities. My kind of doctor.

But I still needed a second opinion. I followed him to the nurses' station where he obtained Dr. B.'s number. I thanked him, and we left.

On the way to the car, I did my usual self-pep talk to dilute the rising fears. *I can handle this. A loss of hearing in one ear. Not so bad. Possible temporary facial weakness. Doesn't sound so terrible. Small risk of stroke. Should not be a problem for me. I'm in good health. At least I don't have cancer.*

Over the next few weeks, I pondered my past, present, and future, my sickness and health. What a year! My sullied sabbatical was coming to a close, and the internal pressure to bring home some Morning Star Breakfast Strips was starting to erupt. Daydreams of re-employment formed a healthy sidebar to moderate the ever-growing fears of the impending surgery.

I updated my résumé and placed it on file at one of the few employers in Nashville large enough to provide medical coverage *without* excluding preexisting conditions—Vanderbilt. As a four-time cancer winner, I did not want to risk losing my state-sponsored insurance plan for low-income or uninsurable Tennesseans.

1998, SEPTEMBER

One Saturday morning in September, I was awakened with the perfect call. An acquaintance and professional colleague, Barbara, had seen my résumé on file and was calling to inquire about my interest in a job as director of a mentoring program for pregnant women and young mothers living in impoverished communities. The program was called the Maternal Infant Health Outreach Worker Project (MIHOW). The new director would be guiding the future of this network of programs in four states as well as expanding the services into two new states.

Bingo! It was the right job for me and my skills. Both Barbara and I intuitively knew this match needed no exotic courting dance. But was it the right time?

The following Monday, I met with Barbara and Mary, the current director, for the formal interview. Toward the end of the interview, I revealed my latest looming handicap. "As good a match as this seems for both me and MIHOW, I have a health problem that may preclude me from the job. I was diagnosed with a brain tumor and will be having surgery next month. I've been told it's very unlikely to be cancerous, but the surgery is pretty major. I'm not sure how long it will take me to recover, but I'm guessing it will be several weeks, possibly even longer, before I'd be able to start."

Much to my surprise, they looked at each other and shrugged their shoulders. "No problem. We're willing to wait."

Then Mary said, "What kind of brain tumor is it, if you don't mind me asking?"

"It's called an acoustic neuroma—they think. They won't know for sure until they get in there. I actually don't know a whole lot about it yet, but an acoustic neuroma is a pretty rare tumor of the hearing and balance nerve. I may be deaf in my right ear afterward."

Mary looked startled. "You're not going to believe this, but I think my neighbor Tom had that kind of tumor a couple of years ago. He seems to be getting along well now. Would you like to talk with him?"

"Sure. I've not talked with anyone yet who has had this kind of tumor, and I'm just now trying to figure out when and where to have the surgery. Talking with someone who has actually been through the surgery would be very helpful."

I left with his name and number and a giddiness about the prospects of a new job to look forward to after the surgery. Despite the ruin of my year off, I was antsy to delve into someone else's problems and to get paid again for something I could do well.

As soon as I got home, I called Tom's number, introduced myself and my reason for calling, then asked if he had time to talk.

"Sure," Tom said. "I don't know if I can be of any help, but I'll try."

I launched right in. "Was your brain tumor actually an acoustic neuroma?"

"Yes, it was. I had it removed about three years ago by Dr. S. Is there anything in particular you're interested in?"

"I'm not really sure. I guess I'm interested in knowing more about what the surgery was like. How did you feel afterward?"

"Do you want to know the truth?" he asked rather ominously.

"Yes. Please tell me what it was like. I've had a lot of surgeries, so I'm no stranger to these kinds of experiences."

He paused. "Well, after the surgery, I wished I were dead."

Silence.

More silence.

"Sorry," he said. "You said you wanted the truth."

Bam! Suddenly, in that distant, yet oh-too-close space where the heart meets the brain, SOS signals were firing. I took in a calming breath. "Thank you. Knowing the truth will help me prepare. Tell me more. What was so bad?"

"I had excruciating headaches. They lasted almost a year. It was awful."

Once he started recounting his saga, there was no turning back. "Another man here on campus, a faculty member in the Owen School of Management, had headaches even worse than mine. He had to give himself shots of morphine. Once, we were walking across campus, and his pain got so bad, he had to stop right then and go give himself a shot."

Another span of silence.

"Everyone's story is different," he said. "Have you been in touch with the Acoustic Neuroma Association?"

"No, I've never heard of them." I should have guessed. There are support groups for everyone, even a support group for support groups, as Barry says.

"You should check out their Web site and newsletters. They have chat rooms where people share stories."

"I'll do that. Thanks. How are you feeling now? Are you still having headaches?"

"Not very often anymore. And when I do, they are much milder."

"That's good to hear. At least they eventually go away. I've had a lot of stuff done to my body, but this is a whole new ball game, and you've given me some important information. Thank you so much for talking with me *and* for being so forthright. Do you mind if I call you again if other questions come to mind?"

"Sure. Anytime. I hope I didn't say too much."

"Oh, no. You've been incredibly helpful."

"Well, good luck, Minda."

"Thank you, Tom."

I hung up the phone and did the usual. I froze. My body was stuck to the chair by a Super Glue of terror. Then my mind went blank. I felt nothing. I was nothing. Just there. Not there.

After a few minutes, I stood up and moved on autopilot. I walked down the stairs and into Barry's office. I turned on his computer, fixated on the blank screen, listened to the modem sing its slow, repetitious tune while dialing up.

I typed "acoustic neuroma" into the Netscape search program, then clicked on the first choice listed, assuming I was headed to the Web site of the Acoustic Neuroma Association. Up popped a chat room with a long chronicle of stories dating back a couple of years. I read the first story. In graphic detail, a woman shared her nightmare of debilitating headaches, nauseating imbalance, facial paralysis, extreme exhaustion, additional surgeries . . .

I read the next story. Then the next. And the next. Two hours later, I could read no more. Acoustic neuromas were obviously dangerous terrorists in benign disguise. And the surgery was the tumor's accomplice to wreak havoc on your world.

When Barry walked in from an environmental consulting gig, I was still staring at the computer. He came into the office and plopped down on the sofa. "What's for dinner?"

"ARE YOU CRAZY?" I yelled. "WHAT'S FOR DINNER? WHAT'S FOR DINNER?"

I was so frantic, I just kept yelling. "I'm facing major brain surgery that's going to leave me with crippling headaches, deafness, a screwed up face, and who knows what else. And you're asking what's for dinner? Don't you have an ounce of sympathy?"

"Uh, sorry."

Barry had walked into a trap, oblivious to the tales of horror I had just read. I was ready to leap across the room and strangle him. Of course he was not the problem, but who else could I strangle? My boxy plastic computer was not pliable enough to crush.

Then the shamed, puppy-dog look on Barry's face broke through my misplaced anger. Bye bye, Dr. Jekyll. Hello, Ms. Hyde.

"Man, I'm sorry," I told him. "You had no way of knowing what I've been through over the past couple of hours." Then I divulged the gist of my conversation with Tom and the sad stories I found.

He quickly put the anecdotes into perspective. "We may be in for more than we bargained for, but remember, people who have good outcomes usually don't tell their stories in a chat room. They get on with their lives. We need to talk with Dr. Jackson again and see what he has to say."

A voice of calm once again. My soul mate. Where would I be without him? Barry helped me climb out of the nightmare and grab a clarifying breath of fresh air. We went into the kitchen to make dinner.

Sure enough, I soon discovered that I had not even been looking at the Acoustic Neuroma Association's Web site. Instead, I had accidentally wandered into a chat room of misery and lament. Grieving can be a *very* important step for recovering patients, but it's not at all helpful to the uninitiated.

I also learned Tom's headaches were probably the result of a procedure rarely used anymore. Dr. Jackson had briefly mentioned but discarded this procedure. I called Uncle Stanley, the retired anesthesiologist living in LA, to access some of his love and advice. He had already talked with my mother, tracked the LA doc grapevine to the famous Dr. B., and contacted him. Dr. B. was expecting a call from me.

No time to waste. I picked up the phone and dialed Dr. B.'s number. He was in surgery, so the receptionist offered to take a message.

"This is Minda Lazarov, an acoustic neuroma patient in Nashville, Tennessee. I've been referred by Dr. Gary Jackson and Dr. Stanley Saperstein."

"I'll be glad to give him the message. What's your number?"

As I gave her my number, I thought, *how many days it will be before I hear from him?*

Within an hour, he called back. I was speechless, wondering what my uncle or I had said to produce this remarkable response time.

"Thank you so much for calling me back," I said. "I was told you are *The* Man I need to talk with about my acoustic neuroma."

I told him my story, and he patiently listened as if he were sitting in a fishing boat, with all the time in the world, waiting for a catch.

When I finished, he asked, "Have you lost any hearing in your right ear?"

"I don't think so. I haven't noticed any change in my hearing."

"Do this for me. Hold the phone up to your right ear."

I did as he instructed. "Can you hear me?"

"Yes. Not a problem."

"This is good. You may be a candidate for the middle fossa approach to remove the tumor. Did Dr. Jackson mention this type of surgery to you?"

"Yes, he did briefly, but we didn't discuss it much. What's it called again?"

"Fossa. Middle fossa."

"Yes. I remember. He said the middle fossa approach might preserve my hearing. How is it different from the translab?"

"We go in above your ear. By entering from this angle, we're able to go around the middle and inner ear and hopefully leave the acoustic nerve intact, thereby preserving the hearing. We used to be able to preserve hearing only with smaller tumors, but now we're having pretty good success with some medium-size ones as well. How big is your tumor?"

"It's 2.2 centimeters. It has grown the entire length of the cerebellopontine angle, from the inner ear to the brain stem."

"A 2.2-centimeter tumor is almost at the upper limit for the middle fossa surgery. But if most of your hearing is still intact, we should have a pretty good chance of preserving it."

"Wow. I was getting accustomed to the idea of hearing loss. This is a lot to think about. I'll talk with my husband. We may have additional questions. Is it okay if I call you back?"

"Sure. If I'm in surgery, I'll return your call afterward."

Who said knowledge is power? I had more knowledge than ever about the surgical point of entry into my brain to escort out my pesky intruder, yet I was more baffled than ever. To translab or middle fossa? *Fossa* sounded more gentle than *translab*. Drilling a path through the middle fossa as opposed to the labyrinth struck me as less invasive, even though I had no idea what and where the fossa was. The House Ear Clinic and Dr. B. were the most well-known names in AN surgery. Yet Dr. Jackson also was at the top of the international list. How was I to decide?

To superimpose order on the chaos whirling in my defective brain, I identified four questions to be answered to help make this decision:

1. Which method had the fewest risks?
2. How debilitating would one-eared hearing be?
3. Was there sufficient evidence that Dr. B. was a better surgeon than Dr. Jackson, and if so, what would it be like to recover two thousand miles from home?
4. If your wife had this tumor, which method would you recommend?

Several conversations later with both Dr. Jackson and Dr. B., I finished the game of Medical Maze with a reasonable dose of confidence. Dr. Jackson would perform the AN-ectomy via the translab approach in the Baptist Operating Room in Nashville.

It had taken several weeks to dig through the clues, but eventually the evidence pointed in a single direction. Here's how the clues were distilled down to a final answer:

Clue 1: The translab approach would enable the surgeon to see most clearly the pathway to the tumor, the tumor itself, and the brain stem. This least obstructed view would allow for the greatest likelihood of reacting most speedily and effectively to the unexpected, such as a blood clot or a bloody, messy mass clinging to the facial nerve that might need extracting piece by piece.

Clue 2: Loss of hearing in one ear, caused by the translab approach, would destroy my ability to discern sound direction and to comprehend group speak at cocktail parties. On the other hand, there was no guarantee the middle fossa method would preserve my hearing. Worse, that method might not completely eliminate the tumor, so the likelihood of a recurrence would be higher.

Clue 3: The thought of waking up from surgery in LA, far from my loved ones in Nashville, was troubling. Though I relished the vision of the loving, supportive Saperstein clan by my bedside, the California location posed another problem as well. Could I sit on a plane for the four-hour return flight to Tennessee? Envisioning a plane ride while I battled post-surgery pain, discomfort, and exhaustion left me a little queasy.

Clue 4: This deal-breaker clue did not emerge until I asked Dr. B. the billion-dollar question: "If your wife had this tumor, which method would you recommend?"

Dr. B. had been the primary cheerleader for the middle fossa approach, but when I asked that question, without a millisecond hesitation, he answered, "Translab."

I was stunned. "Why?"

It turned out that the size of my tumor and the additional risk of a stroke did not warrant an attempt to save my hearing in one ear. It took me a while to understand how the detour to the middle fossa had occurred. It was my mistake. I'd given Dr. B. the impression that my hearing was a top priority, while in actuality, my preference was to get through this ordeal with the fewest complications and least risk of recurrence. Period. All other concerns were a distant second.

Clue 5: Once I knew translab was *the* surgical approach of choice, the final question was, who should perform the surgery, Dr. Jackson or Dr. B.? Additional research revealed I would be in good hands either way, with a surgeon who had been inside hundreds of skulls, seen hundreds of situations, and had hundreds of opportunities to experience those odd situations. Dr. Jackson had one up on Dr. B., however. He was two thousand miles closer. Dr. Jackson was my man.

At the same time I was making these decisions, I was also priming my body and mind. This surgery was not an ambush, so I had plenty of time to prepare for the battle. I relied on the triple whammy of my loosely defined religious faith, my scientific training and research, and Tom Hanks.

Mr. Hanks was in Nashville filming the movie *The Green Mile* at the historic, abandoned Tennessee State Penitentiary near our house. I love Tom Hanks. What better time to make a case for a personal meet-and-greet than when I was on the rebound from breast cancer and gearing up for brain tumor surgery? So I wrote him a letter.

I explained to him my dire predicament. I had been through four bouts of cancer, six major surgeries, and massive doses of radiation and chemotherapy. I began the year with breast cancer and was finishing it off with a slash-and-burn attack inside my skull. What better way to enter surgery in the most positive frame of mind than to get a bear hug from my favorite actor? One minute, one hug. *Please?*

Barry, Shea, her best friend, Savannah, and I drove up to the back of the hundred-year-old turreted castle as the sun was setting. We were on a mission to sneak into the gated fortress and find someone who would deliver my plea to Tom. The guard stopped us at the entrance. He wasn't buying the story. I was ready to leap out of the car, pull up my blouse, and show him my mounds and abdominal scars, but the boss man Barry said no. So I handed the letter to the guard, and Barry turned the car around and drove away.

I later mailed a copy of the letter to the Tennessee Film Commission, asking them to deliver it to Tom, hoping he might at least visit me in the hospital.

I waited for the call. And I waited.

I held onto the vision of a Hanks Hug until the day of the surgery. I dreamed Tom appeared at my bedside as I was saying my last good-byes before being wheeled off to the OR.

I never heard from Tom. Twerp.

As for the other components of my surgery prep, Rabbi Kanter always referred to the Sh'ma as the watchwords of our Jewish faith. I recited this prayer every day: "Sh'ma Yisrael Adonai Eloheinu . . ." I interpreted the Sh'ma not literally, but rather as a long mantra that stirred a faith-based hope in my skeptical psyche. I read the Sh'ma out loud, softly to myself, and the Hebrew words reverberated from within and without. This powerful prayer merged physical vibrations and spiritual awakenings to create an immediate source of strength.

With the door to my Judaism opened, I accessed another potent Jewish practice where orthodoxy met alternative medicine. Barry and I were introduced to healing touch, Kabbalah style, by Barry's cousin Mark. Initially I was shocked when my religiously scarred, New Age husband consented to participate in this faith-based healing expedition, but we both were reaching for any possible help to boost my sagging body and spirit. We drove to Mark and Sandy's home in Louisville to seek guidance from his mystical wisdom.

Mark provided a crash course in a few basic Kabbalistic tenets. We learned the two-hundred-forty-eight Hebrew words of the Sh'ma corresponded to the two-hundred-forty-eight segments of the soul and body. Furthermore, the order and sounds of the Hebrew letters and words carried healing power. These interpretations helped me bridge the gap between the meaningless English translations and the profound impact the prayer had had on me over several decades.

To access Barry's love and healing powers, Mark taught Barry a Jewish version of healing touch, and upon our return to Nashville, Barry performed this daily ritual, the laying on of hands as he recited a Hebrew prayer. Also, Mark described crying as a direct connection to the soul, helping to explain why it felt spiritually uplifting to cry, regardless of the degree of sadness or joy.

As with the previous ordeals, I continued researching what in the heck was about to happen so I could help dissolve my fear of the unknown. By studying the anatomical details of the skull, ear, and tumor location, I was able to conjure up a productive mental image. My mind's eye could zoom in on the cozy little spot where my tumor was napping so my bristled brushes could whittle the rascal down.

I also read the quintessential textbook on how to snip away an acoustic neuroma, Dr. House's *Translabyrinthine Approach: Otologic Surgery*. From this book, I learned about the layers of matter the surgeons would traverse to get to the tumor.

As a first step, the assisting surgeons would cut a C-shaped incision behind and paralleling the curve of my right ear. This slice would allow them to peel back the ear and move the thin layer of connective tissue called the fascia out of the way to expose the skull. Next, using a mighty fine diamond bit, they would drill a one-inch hole in my skull, then cut an opening in the leathery dura encasing my brain (sort of like a thick-skinned Polish sausage). Each tool could be passed through this hole as needed. Finally, they would strip-mine the area to uncover the ugly chunk of coal. Bye bye, mastoid bone, middle ear bones, and cochlea. Finally, after about four hours of surgery, they would call in Dr. Jackson.

Depending on whether I had propagated a good guy or a bad guy, Dr. Jackson would stretch, fray, or cut away the facial nerve (VII) from the acoustic/balance nerve (VIII), along with neighbors VI and IX. His goal would be to isolate the acoustic nerve and the tumor so he could cut them out with minimal collateral damage. The amount of damage depended on just how closely the tumor had snuggled up to its neighbors.

After Dr. Jackson removed the tumor, he would open my belly, again at the site of the ovarian surgery and faux nipple extraction, then slice out a piece of fat and slip it into the place where the mastoid bone had been. Lastly, he would seal the dura and gently reattach the useless ear, taking care to align it with the good one. That was it!

Fully visualizing how the surgeons would approach, capture, and destroy the enemy had two very positive outcomes. First, these details allowed me to practice meditation and mental imagery in a more focused way. This knowledge also increased my confidence in Dr. Jackson and his team, the surgery itself, and the outcome, whatever it might bring. As a result, I was able to rest deeply in the nights leading up to the surgery and to maintain a sense of peace in the final hour as I was prepped to have a hole drilled into my head.

1998, OCTOBER

On October 26, 1998, I checked into Baptist Hospital. We had eighteen hours until showtime with a busy pre-surgical VIP schedule. At the request of Dr. Jackson, Barry and I made the rounds to meet each member of the surgical team. We felt like political lobbyists soliciting support for our upcoming bill.

That evening, Barry, Shea, and I left the hospital for the Last Supper with Mom and Dad at the Noshville

Deli. After dinner we said our good-byes and retreated
to the hospital room. Joe, our good friend, ordained
minister, and death row inmate counselor, came by and
led us through a group prayer. Then we formed a
huddle as Joe made a valiant attempt to get the three of
us talking about our fears and hopes. We were
speechless. None of us had the stoutness of spirit to
verbalize our emotions. His prayer was much needed,
though, as we desperately held onto each other,
wishing the next day could be snatched off the
calendar.

Shea eventually fell asleep. Barry moved her into
the other bed, and then the two of us drifted off,
hugging each other as tightly as possible—as if this was
our last night together.

I was awakened at 4:00 a.m. and told to get into the
shower and wash my hair with Phisohex. I wanted to
ask, "Do you have Nexxus Therappe instead?" Though
Phisohex would make my hair dry and stringy, I quietly
took the green plastic bottle from the nurse, got in the
shower, and turned on the water as hot as I could bear
it. The warmth helped to wash away my fears.

The day is finally here, I thought, *and everything is out
of my hands. I've got a fabulous surgeon, husband, daughter,
mother, and father by my side and lots of love blowing my
way from my sister and dozens of other friends and family.
Let's get the show on the road.*

Next thing I remember, I woke up in the neuro-
Intensive Care Unit. There I stayed for three days. Barry
and Shea were the first of my loved ones to see me. I
don't remember their visit, but Shea does. It is burned
into her memory forever. She put the memory on paper
three years later as part of an English assignment.

The Ring Bearer
by Shea Sulkin
[written at age sixteen,
three years after the acoustic neuroma surgery]

The most important wedding of my life, but I am not wearing the dress. I sit in my cold, hard chair waiting for the moment when I set my eyes on the bride. The anticipation rises in my body and I question wether [*sic*] the bride will make it to her own ceremony. How upset we would all be at this wedding without a bride. But the music stops, and the ceremony starts. The bride has finally arrived.

She is dressed from head to knee in her bridal gown. Her head is asymmetrically wrapped in a veil of white gauze to cover her imperfections. Instead of the cumbersome and seemingly unnecessary train from her dress, she wears tubes from her arms. And at this wedding, there are no bridesmaids, no best men, no flower girls, no ring bearers here. Or, perhaps I am the bearer of the ring, only it isn't a ring on a red, velvet cushion. I carry my sunken heart, and my heart is what keeps the bride alive. I can't bear to keep my chin up knowing that my heart has fallen down to my stomach, pulling with it tears of pain. I wish to drag all the hurt from her body, because she is not deserving of it. But in turn, all I can do is press together my lips and simulate a smile as if it were real, because this truly is the happiest moment of my life. She tries to smile at me to let me know the worst is over, but I already know. Every nerve in my body is shaking to tell me that she's fine. I know there is no need to worry because she is Superwoman to me, and Superwoman has no fear.

I stand there, staring with my father. I want to grab her into my arms and hold her tight, but I'm pushed away. Pushed by the stale, clean smell of her hospital room and the dark lighting to hide her scars. The rhythmic beeping of her life line drives me farther away with each beep, beep, beep. My father's expression holds me back. I have never seen such suffering strike across his strong face. I bite my dry, tasteless tongue and repress my wails and cries of anguish. Instead of pulling her into my arms, I squeeze my sweaty palms so tight that the salty liquid drips from my bloodless knuckles. I hold it all in to hide my disheartening emotions from her. I want her to see my young strength, but I can barely find any courage.

She slowly lifts her heavy eyelids, and as if it has been rehearsed again and again, she remarks, "At least I can smile." The sharp pain of happiness hits my heart and radiates to my toes and my temples. A true smile slides across my face as I slowly turn letting the tears run from my eyes. I walk away from this moment knowing I was once her miracle, but now she is mine. Instead of a ring on the red, velvet cushion, I brought this bride a gift better than diamonds and gold. I brought the gift of eternal love to my mother's marriage with life.

chapter fourteen

1998, OCTOBER

The eternal love Shea spoke of in her tender story kept our nuclear unit afloat during my three days in intensive care. The excruciating angst and sensitivity Shea experienced at that first sighting of her mauled mother infused in her young adolescent psyche a mature outlook on health, sickness, and the composite of the two we call life. With this inchoate wisdom came strength—as well as a few medical phobias—but that's another story.

Barry also was jolted by the sight of me, but he managed to recover. He had plenty of experience observing my ability to pull through and recuperate, which led to a somewhat naïve assumption that I could do it again—and again—and again.

My journey was easiest during the three days in ICU. If I felt fear, pain, or loss of control, I don't remember it. The part of my brain in charge of short-term memory must have been impaired because I recall little about the ICU stay, conceivably a blessing in disguise. Or maybe Dr. Jackson and his cronies used a secret trick to erase my memories of postsurgical trauma.

By the time they wheeled me away to a private hospital room, I was cognizant of only two brief events during the three days in ICU. Both memories left vivid imprints so I can still call them up like a YouTube clip.

I'm in the full recumbent position on the gurney. My eyes are closed. My eyes are open. Where am I? I can hear before I can see. The familiar electronic beep, beep, beep, common in scenes from *ER*, sparked this first moment of awareness.

"Mrs. Lazarov?" I recognize that voice. My head turns to the left, ever so slowly and deliberately, just far enough to catch a blurred, double vision image of a large girth between the chrome bars of the gurney.

"Everything went very well, Mrs. Lazarov."

Ah, yes. Dr. Jackson. I cannot see his face. My view from the gurney includes only the fuzzy outline of his torso in a blue surgical gown. I talk to his waist, intuitively knowing he will talk back. My words are slurred, barely audible.

"Was it . . . a good guy . . . or a bad guy?"

"It was not a good guy. We got it out, though, and you're doing fine." (Later, when I was no longer flat on my back, he disclosed that he'd had to remove it piece by piece like a "wet Kleenex.")

Sometime during the next hour, the next day, the next night, I have no idea—I awoke again, desperately yearning to move my head. Blazing across the storyboard of my battered brain were dreadful testimonies from acoustic neuroma patients of the misery generated by traumatized head and neck muscles. Despite my determined will, I could barely nudge my head in any direction.

"Aaahhhhhh," I whimpered. "Aaahhhhhhhh . . . heeelllp."

A floating, faceless, female voice spoke. "What can I do for you?"

"Would you . . . please . . . turn my . . . my head . . . . to the side?"

She obliged, gently cradling both sides of my head with her hands as she turned it to the left, away from the disaster site. My eyes drifted shut. The crisis was over. End of memory. Sometime later, same memory. Later, same memory again.

My next recollection was waking up in a private hospital room on the neurosurgical floor. I guess I'd been recently transported from the ICU, and deposited in my new bed. I regained consciousness in a semi-upright, slumped position. Eyes closed. Eyes open. The wooden cross on the wall at the end of my bed came into focus.

I turned my head to the right. Sitting in the chair next to the bed was Wendy Kanter, the rabbi's wife, with a red clown's nose planted on the middle of her face. It was Halloween, October 31, 1998. Her model perfect, Julia Roberts's smile instantaneously flicked on my one-sided, half-crescent acoustic neuroma smile. (The other half of my smile got left in the OR.)

As I write this, I still have the red sponge nose, though I don't have Wendy, except in my heart. She died of breast cancer in 2007.

I have Rebecca, though. That evening, she stood at the side of my bed and told my other visitors, "Minda just had brain surgery, and she still looks beautiful."

It's hard to imagine a pale-faced, gauze-turbanized, war-torn soldier just back from the front lines as beautiful, but I believed her.

No other memories survived those remaining two days in the hospital. No other flashes of food, family, or friends are retrievable. The events of those days are lost to the dark crevices of the cerebrum where drug- and trauma-induced memories hide.

When I got home, a reconnaissance of the surgery's effects revealed the twitching eyelid was gone. The imaginary sensation of saliva hanging on my lip was gone. The lightheadedness was gone. The collateral damage was widespread, however. Hearing in my right ear was gone, but silence did not step into the void. Rather, my unilateral deafness gave birth to the constant whirring of a phantom Eureka vacuum cleaner.

The noise has not stopped for a millisecond since. It has a back beat any jazz lover might appreciate. Amidst the background of the incessant electric static is a bang, bang, pause, bang, pause, bang, bang, bang. It's got the beat of a non-terminating number, sort of like pi, with no repetitions. Or maybe I just haven't concentrated long enough to detect the pattern. Now there's a useful goal. Perhaps some esoteric truth about the meaning of life is hidden in the measure of the beats.

Then there was the dripless tear duct and semi-catatonic eyelid that would not shut all the way. My blinker was on the blink. With no tears and a lengthened exposure to dry air and debris from the lazy eyelid, my eye required supplemental moisture. I'd always been foreign-matter-in-the-eye challenged, so

Barry had to wrestle with me to lie still while he directed the singular drop from the tiny torture bottle onto my cornea. I eventually got the hang of it and was able to self-lubricate.

To protect the exposed eyeball while I slept, I taped a clear plastic dome over my eye. The nifty, shallow, bowl-shaped ophthalmologic aid looked like the topside of the packaging for a Silly Putty egg. The key feature was a quarter-inch, flat outer edge with an adhesive strip for adhering the cup to the face. The adhesive conveniently worked for just one application, two if you were lucky. Three dollars multiplied by countless naps and evenings did not add up to a new Lexus, but the sum would surely fill up the tank a few times. Since I had no idea how long I would need the contraption, I reused each cup for at least seven days and nights by attaching it in place with surgical tape.

The regular dose of viscous eye drops hampered my 20/20 vision. I could decipher faces and read, albeit slowly, by moving my forefinger from line to line. But threading a needle was difficult. Ava reported her most vivid caretaker memory of Surgery Number Eight was Minda sitting up in bed at home, hemming a dress for Shea. Matching the end of a thread to the eye of a needle was not going to stop this mother from making darn sure the hem of her daughter's dress was *exactly* six inches above the knee to simmer down the pre-party teen jitters.

The next stop on this tour of the injuries was a frayed and swollen facial nerve too frazzled to communicate with the brain. As a result, the muscles on the right side of my face went into a deep sleep (hence, the crippled eyelid). Technically speaking, I scored six out of seven on the paralysis scale, indicating a modicum of juice remained in my facial nerve. I could not feel or see *any* facial movement on the right, however. No forehead wrinkles, no squinting, no scrunching of the nose, no upturn of the lips, nothing.

Upon first glance, my smile created an immediate dissonance for the viewer. With none of the normal tugging from the traumatized *right* side to balance the fully functioning muscles on the *left* side, my face yielded two extremely contrasting expressions—an overly happy face on the left and a deer-in-the-headlights glare on the right. People would gaze at me, trying to figure out which side was faulty. Most folks wrongly assumed the damage was on the crazed clown side. It took a few months, but I finally got used to the furtive glances of strangers.

My stunned facial muscles also wreaked havoc on the most fine-tuned skill Americans share in common—eating. My chewing, tasting, swallowing, and sucking mechanisms were significantly impaired. With a broken sucker, I could no longer make a seal with my lips and, therefore, could not suck on a straw or drink neatly from a glass. Saliva escaped in unsightly dribbles down my chin.

Then there was the greatly hampered movement of the right side of the tongue. Try this. Take a hefty bite of a peanut butter and jelly sandwich, and let it land on the right side of your tongue. Now try and chew it without moving your tongue. Next try and move it toward your throat in preparation for the swallow without moving your tongue.

Movement of the tongue is one of those precious, involuntary responses we fail to appreciate. *Thank you, tongue, for your devoted work ethic all these years.*

So I learned the art of one-sided mastication. If I failed to stay focused and a morsel of food slid over to the right side of my tongue, I had to reach in with my fingers to push it over to the working side. On occasion, the food just fell out of my mouth before I had a chance to retrieve it. In truth, though, I had no real desire to masticate on the right side anyway—the taste buds were also asleep at the wheel.

Next on the list of collateral damage was my lower lip. Normally when you bite a sandwich, your lower lip automatically skirts out of the way of harm. But when you paralyze the lower lip muscles, an innocent bite of turkey sandwich can lead to a bloody altercation.

And then there was the weakened nerve which controlled my swallowing muscle. Lord help me when I had a hankering for a hunk of meat. It was more than my abused swallower could handle. Until I finally learned my limits, I sometimes resorted to sticking my fingers into the back of my mouth to yank out the chewed ball of meat, divide it in two and try again.

Between the tongue handicap and the loose lips, I was not a well-sought-after dinner guest. Of course my hairdo didn't help either. A third of my head had been shaved, revealing a six-inch C-shaped line of staples behind my ear. Twenty hours of daily sleepy time, with no attempt to bring order with a comb, twisted the remaining two-thirds of my long wavy mane into a mess of matted hair as ghastly as Mrs. Frankenstein's coiffure.

To complete the pitiful picture, the swelling made the top of my ear stick out twenty degrees. Alfalfa from the *Little Rascals* didn't hold a candle to my goofy look. And we're not finished yet. Hang in there with me, and you will soon have the complete image.

Drilling through the skull and cutting through the leathery dura encasing the brain can sometimes lead to a spinal fluid leak. Usually, when this happens, the fluid chooses the nose as the exit route, causing an intense headache. I'd experienced something like this before, and I wanted no more of it. So I followed an obligatory rule of limited motion: do not bend over below the waist.

I had heard horror stories from AN patients who got antsy and wandered out to their abandoned gardens too soon. One patient claimed the mishap occurred almost a year after her surgery. She got too ambitious pulling weeds and bent over one too many times. Whisssh. Out poured the spinal fluid from her nose onto her newly planted snapdragons. Dr. Jackson had to surgically go back into the skull and seal up the leak. I was scared into submission by these stories and became a fanatic about the perils of dipping my head below the waist.

The most significant alteration was detectable by only Barry, Shea, and me. An avalanche of fatigue. The word *extreme* is not extreme enough. My life force had been yanked out of me. In all my exposures to surgery, radiation, and chemotherapy, I had never known this degree of languor. I felt the weariness at a subcellular level, as though my cells had absolutely no reserve of energy, and even the tiniest movements of body or mind pushed me farther into the red.

So I slept and slept. I woke up long enough to carefully spoon some nourishment into the left side of my mouth. And to read. For six weeks, there was nothing to do but eat, sleep, and read. It was divine.

Each morning after a night of deep sleep and a leisurely breakfast, I nestled my disabled self into my favorite stuffed chair from Goldsmith's Department store in Memphis. Green and mauve roses surrounded the deer standing in the open pasture of the well-padded seat and back. There I sat, hour after hour, focusing my altered vision, stopping only to moisten my dry eye and offer relief to one of the few unaltered body parts—my bladder.

I read a trilogy on the African-American journey while sitting in that chair: *Cloudsplitter*, a fictional tale of John Brown; *Walking with the Wind*, the memoir of Congressman John Lewis; and *Thurgood Marshall: An American Revolutionary*, a biography of the first black Supreme Court justice. Every hour or so, my head fell back on a green rose, and I drifted off. Sleep was always seconds away. The need to sleep clung to me.

In the aftermath of my previous seven surgeries, music had been a runner-up to sleep as a powerful healing agent. The sounds of music from the Beatles, Jackson Browne, Nanci Griffith and Bonnie Raitt had always instilled a welcomed comfort that shot straight to the places that needed attention. Eventually, the Grateful Dead at high volume became an energizing accompaniment to cooking, writing, cleaning house—

those tasks were a surefire sign I was on the road to recovery.

Not this time. The sensory changes from the surgery altered my reaction to music. Too many decibels or high notes made my spine crawl. Most all music at any level made me squirm. The combination of music and other background noise, even a simple hum of a computer, generated an irritation similar to nails being dragged across a chalkboard.

There were a couple of exceptions, however. The melodious sound waves of the harp played by my dear and talented friend Kathleen were as healing as a trip to the beach. Something about the harp, and the harpist, resonated through my tired body, reconnecting disjointed energy pathways and worn nerves. She hauled her forty-pound spruce and mahogany harp up the hill and into my living room to pluck old English, Irish, and Yiddish tunes. Golden-toned vibrations drifted into my supine body as I stretched out on the sofa like Cleopatra.

Jonell Mosser's songs were another effective musical elixir. Her album *So Like Joy* made me get up and dance. Often when I was home alone, I placed Jonell's CD in the slot, and as soon as the introductory notes of "Parasite" bellowed out of the speakers, I was out of the chair, my arms outstretched, body slowly— very slowly because my balance was fragile—twirling in slender figure eights. Or I closed my eyes, gently rocking in place and weeping as she sang "So Like Joy," a tribute to her deceased mother. By the time I got to the last song, based on an traditional Irish prayer, called "Blessing," I was in a blissful state.

May the rain always fall
    Soft upon your fields
And the sun pour down like honey
    Where you stand.
May the wind be at your back
    And the road rise to meet you
And your soul rest at last
    In the hollow of God's hands.
Life isn't easy.
No one ever said it was.

—"Blessing"

Sparks of joy radiated outward from my fatigued body and soul as I swirled around the furniture, feeling Jonell's song of gratitude lifting me higher (schmaltzy, but true). And this was without drugs. Amazing what an earnest beating can do for the soul.

The most surprising postsurgical event was the most uplifting of all. I had no headaches! Not one, not even for one fleeting moment. In fact, despite all of the fracases, I had no pain! The credit for this miracle landed right in the laps of Dr. Jackson and his stellar surgical team.

The absence of pain translated into motivation to fix the broken parts, and numerous creative interventions were suggested to mend my damaged goods. To get the blinker working again, my ophthalmologist offered an outpatient surgery to insert a small gold weight in my eyelid to help it close. I declined. With a drained reservoir of energy, the thought of another physical trauma, no matter how small, was incomprehensible. Dr. Jackson understood my story as if he had been there himself, and as soon as I asked his advice, he said patience would probably lead to the same outcome. Instead, an innocuous tiny silicone plug was placed in the corner of my eye to conserve the naturally produced tears.

As the days rolled by, my energy gradually improved, and I began to wash a few dishes, fold a few towels, pick up a broom. I was always mindful, however, of not bending over, calling out for Shea or Barry to fetch the dust pan. Barry never tired of coming to my aid to help build my strength. He demonstrated his concern by acquiring for me a professional-style dust pan with a four-foot handle so I could sweep the entire house without bending over.

A genuine sign of feeling better is some small gesture of concern about one's physical appearance. A couple of weeks after the surgery, the staples and gauze turban were removed. Without these props, I looked like a Dick Tracy character. I have to admit, at first I relished the freakish facade and the response it solicited. Yes, ma'am, I wanted some respect for my battle wounds.

One Saturday morning, I woke up and crawled downstairs for Barry's energy-boosting breakfast— homemade waffles, yogurt, OJ, and coffee. I plodded back upstairs, grabbed my toothbrush, and applied one small squirt of Crest creamy blue. When I looked into the mirror, I was stunned by the monster staring back at me. I resembled a drugged-out homeless lady who had not come in contact with tools of hygiene in many moons. Evidently the unfortunate woman had survived a knife fight that left a prominent red C–shaped slash around her ear.

I could not take my eyes off the disturbing image. By the time I was finished cleansing my half smile, I had decided that shaving the rest of my head was the best solution. I couldn't imagine untangling the matted knots from my once beautiful hair. A clean shave might freshen my outlook.

Barry and Shea were still sitting at the breakfast table when I reappeared downstairs. They were a little surprised to see me since I usually went back to bed after breakfast.

I said, "I think it's time to shave my head."

In unison they both glared at me and replied emphatically, "No."

I suspected the Sinead O'Conner look would not go over well. "What am I supposed to do then? These knots are not coming out."

Shea said, "Give us a try. Dad and I will see what we can do. Right, Dad?"

That evening, before dinner, Barry brought a kitchen chair without arms into the living room. He moved the floor lamp next to the chair, and I positioned myself comfortably in the padded seat, while Barry and Shea gathered their instruments on a black Formica TV tray. Over the next couple of hours, they took turns *very* patiently working through one knot after another. They were on a mission, a mission I felt sure they would fail because the pain would be intolerable. Yet these hair-combing maestros unraveled each and every knot. I guess the fear of being seen with a hairless freak inspired Barry and Shea with enough patience to complete the task. I metamorphosed from Frankenstein's wife to Frankenstein's mistress. I still looked pretty rough.

Although the hairs were now lying parallel to each other like delinquents beaten into submission, they were dirty, stringy, and in need of love. The last shampoo this hair had known was Phisohex, so after dinner, I washed my hair with my own shampoo.

In our glass-brick shower stall, I sat on an orthopedic shower stool for half an hour, and the continuous stream of hot water across my scalp felt as purifying as a baptism (as best this Jew can know). I was so weak, I could lift my arms only a couple of minutes at a time. By the time I finished, I barely had enough oomph left to wrap my head in a towel and walk the few feet to the bed, where I promptly drifted off.

When I awoke, Shea helped me comb out my hair, a much less challenging chore this time around. I apparently had less patience than she did, though, because Mother and Daughter quarreled with each stroke of the comb.

"Ow, you're hurting me!"

"You're such a wimp! This is what *you* used to do to *me*!"

"Ahhh. The tables are turned, huh? I think you're letting out all your frustrations on me."

"Mom, would you be quiet, please? Stop the psychobabble, and let's just get this over with!"

"Ow, you're hurting me!"

Within a couple of hours, my hair was combed and dried. The extreme makeover had worked. My hair was long and thick enough to cover the naked third of my scalp in a Donald Trumpish comb-over—although I looked a heck of a lot better than Mr. Trump.

I slept hard that night, falling into bed with the exhaustion of a farmer after a day laboring in the hot sun. When I awoke the next morning, I felt a tiny bounce in my feet. Instead of one loop around the yard, I circled the house twice. So began the next phase of the healing journey from Surgery Number Eight. Each day I walked a little farther and slept a little less.

Six weeks after the surgery, Barry insisted I accompany him to a Sierra Club conference in Santa Fe. Prior to the surgery, we had agreed this trip would give me something to look forward to, a target to reach in my crawl toward recovery. I tried to bow out, but Barry wisely insisted I tag along.

At the opening reception, I was greatly humbled as Barry introduced me to one stranger after another. From my previous medical beatings, I knew the role of a woman with a gnarled body. A gnarled face required a different playbook, however. My attempts to laugh or smile produced an expression that was hard for others to look at, and harder to wear. As a former reasonably attractive woman, I suddenly felt a kinship with the aesthetically challenged guests.

The gathering allowed me to test out my new hearing handicap, and the preliminary results were a bit bleak. I had trouble understanding everyone, including the person standing right next to my "good" left ear. Between the cocktail chitter-chatter of people getting to know one another and the vintage Eureka vacuum churning away in the right ear, I could decipher little of the conversation. My brain interpreted the sounds as a string of vague wha-wha-whas, like the gurglings of a toddler. When I was able to pick up discernible words, my brain mangled them. For instance, *Sara's project on the Salmon River* came out sounding like *Sara's object is to maim her.*

As the conferees continued their banter, I felt pressured to access heretofore untapped theatrical talents. I feigned reactions of interest, surprise, or humor, depending on what the others were doing. I'm sure my ten-second delay of an appropriate facial expression conveyed an IQ of about 85. After a while, I politely told the group I felt fatigued from a recent surgery and was going to lie down.

The next day, I ventured out to explore the historic town square of Santa Fe while Barry attended his conference. A short three-block walk to the square seemed doable. Easier said than done with vision, hearing, and balance impairments. My sight was somewhere between single and double vision, sound was a mix between real and distorted, and the ground was neither level nor steady. In the sheltered environment of home, I had sidestepped the reality of these neurological changes, but I could no longer ignore them as I attempted to traverse the icy December sidewalks of Santa Fe. The difficulty of navigating the one-quarter mile of slippery pavement was a bitter-cold slap in my face.

I paced myself, shuffling slowly and methodically across the seemingly high patches of ice until I finally reached the covered walkway of the old cow town center. The former saloons, general store, and stables were now dress, antique, candy, and novelty shops. I sat down at the first bench I came to and caught my breath. Whew! While I was pretty proud of myself for not falling, I was exhausted. My nerves and the senses they controlled were working overtime to keep my body in an upright position.

A brief rest on the bench in the public square renewed my zest for the outing, though my thoughts were thick and ill-formed. I could not congeal words into complete sentences without a determined effort. Yet I felt a strong wave of emotion: *I am frigging lucky to be alive! And here I am still walking (sort of) and talking (sort of)—to myself—not a good sign.*

I got up from the bench and walked into a women's clothing store. The sweaters, dresses, and jewelry perfectly suited my tastes. Usually, I could find something of value anywhere, but I meandered around the store, unable to focus my shopping skills. The saleswoman must have assumed I could walk, see, hear, and think just like anyone else. If I looked up and smiled with my half-frozen face and unique, comb-over hairdo, would she be frightened? I pretended the sweaters I was fondling were clearly visible to me.

"May I help you?" she asked.

"No thank you. Just browsing."

With that brief exchange, I decided it was time to make the long journey home before I passed out on her two-hundred-fifty-year-old, pinewood floor. My fuel indicator was dipping toward empty, and it seemed like miles of ice floe lay between me and the bed. Twenty minutes later, victory was in sight. By the time I got to the room and pulled out the key, I barely had the strength to unlock the door. I went straight for the bed and fell into a deep sleep.

On day three, Barry suggested we check out Bandelier National Monument. This adventure sounded innocent, requiring just enough exertion to lift my spirits. We drove our rental car into the desert about fifty miles outside town. Just past the parking lot, we entered a 1.2-mile walking loop. Halfway around the loop, the trail turned into a twenty-foot, rope-and-log ladder, built Native American style. We had to scale this ladder up the face of a small mesa to finish the loop back to the parking lot.

"Let's go up there," Barry said excitedly. His Eagle Scout sense of adventure had led us on many a wild trek over the years, through creeks, rhododendron thickets, and trackless forests. My trust in his allegiance to his Boy Scout Law to *be trustworthy, loyal, helpful, friendly, courteous, kind, obedient, cheerful, thrifty, brave, clean, and reverent* was not abounding at the moment.

"I don't think so," I pleaded.

"Sure, you can do it. Let's go."

"Nope. Can't do it. Last thing I need right now is to fall and crack my skull. Let's walk back the way we came."

"I'll go right behind you. You can do it. I know you can do it."

"All right. I'll try. But if I get dizzy, we're turning around and heading right back down. Got it?"

"Yes, ma'am. Let's do it."

I grabbed the ladder, pulled myself up to the first rung, and stopped.

"Are you okay?" Barry asked.

"So good, so far," I replied skeptically. I went the next two rungs. "Things are starting to spin."

"I'm right here. Let's keep going."

Two more rungs and then rest, I thought. I made the two rungs and stopped, squeezing the side rails as though I would fall into a thousand-foot chasm if I lost my grip. I took a deep breath, glanced up at the top, scampered up the final rungs, and landed my rump on the icy ground. "I made it!"

"See, I knew you could do it."

In my little world with my one, lone balance nerve, I had just traversed Mt. Kilimanjaro. What mountain could I climb next?

We spent the rest of the afternoon leisurely finishing the loop. Back at the conference center, I stuck to the bed like a fly to flypaper. I slept for several hours, spread out exactly as I had landed. When I awoke, I ventured out to the conference's closing social hour and humbled myself amidst the rugged Sierra Club hikers. It was humiliating to feel like such a lightweight among the hard-core outdoorsmen and women. The next day we flew home, and I slept the entire way back.

The excursion to Santa Fe gave me a glimpse of both the benefits and the challenges I would face as I integrated back into daily social and professional interactions. I returned motivated, yet reluctant, about starting work in a new job. The ambivalence was reflected in my half-paralyzed face. One side of me was all smiles, raring to get back on the horse. The other side was frozen in place, terrified that stress and fatigue might land me back in the claws of the demons. My will to pursue another battle had totally wilted. I was certain one more skirmish could kill me.

While I was preoccupied with the risks and benefits of moving toward normalcy, 1998, the Year from Hell, finally came to a close. Breast cancer, a breastectomy, double mound construction, and intracranial surgery had totally depleted my stamina. Yet I was getting better every day and looking forward to an uneventful 1999!

1999

In January, 1999, the time had arrived to make the leap and return to the land of the gainfully employed. So I became the part-time director of the Maternal Infant Health Outreach Worker Program (MIHOW). I also began teaching nutrition again at the Vanderbilt School of Nursing. By February, three months after the surgery, I decided to dive all the way into a full-time work week. I was very fortunate to have Barbara, a family-and-wellness-friendly boss. She echoed the importance for me to work at home as necessary, and to keep a weekly schedule that rarely exceeded forty hours.

It did not take long to realize the impact of full-time work on my disabled body. Working, feeding, sleeping, and mothering were all I could handle. I awoke at 7:00 a.m., left the house by 8:30, and was home again by 6:00. Sometimes I was so fatigued I would go straight to bed. I tried hard to reserve some energy for Shea, but left most of the parenting to Barry.

A few of my professional responsibilities revealed the depth of the damage. I could not hide my shortcomings as I had done with the previous assaults. Cognitively, I was operating at a deficit in several ways. The most obvious change was in my inability to string together a series of thoughts or concepts to come to a conclusion. It was not a problem of adding four and four and getting ten. I added four and four and got _____. Nothing. Nothing came to mind. When I was fatigued, my brain was unplugged. I became a bumbling idiot. At home, this handicap would drive both Barry and Shea wild.

"What should we have for dinner?" Barry would ask innocently.

"Well . . . look in the . . ."

"Yeeeeeeeees? Look in the what?"

"Look in the fridge. . . . Do we have . . . ?"

"Yes, yes, do we have what?"

"Do we have . . . tomato . . . tomato sauce?"

It might take me several sentences, if ever, to pull together a complete thought. Sometimes I just uncharacteristically replied, "It's up to you and Shea. Whatever you guys want." Like most female heads of households, I usually wanted what I wanted when I wanted it.

Early in my pursuit to force the spent mind and body back into a work schedule, I took a road trip with Mary, my predecessor in the MIHOW director position. She was working a few hours a week during the transition, and I tagged along to participate in an informal training for MIHOW home visitors and to meet some of my new Appalachian colleagues. Six of us gathered around a table in Hazard, Kentucky as Mary led a discussion on finding strengths in disadvantaged families.

Toward the end of the training, Mary turned to me and asked, "Minda, anything you want to add?"

It was late. We had traveled several hours to get there. I had heard parts of the discussion, and I sort of understood her question. But my mind was in a void. I did not want to appear stupid or rude, as though I had not been listening, particularly since part of the training was about listening skills. A first impression as a lackluster dunce was not what any of us had in mind for a new leader.

So I replied, "I agree with everything you said," adding for good measure since I wasn't totally confident in what I was agreeing with, "but I'm unfortunately too tired to add anything helpful to the discussion."

This answer was one of the first of hundreds of attempts to straddle the lines between a dimwit brain tumor victim and a politician. If I took the latter role, I tried my hardest to keep a straight face and make up something that sounded reasonably intelligent, but communicated little of substance.

A mangled body calls for a mangled sense of humor, and once again, Barry stood by to lighten the cosmic load. Whenever I assumed that dumbfounded look as I struggled to interpret what had just been said to me, he jumped in and said, "You have to excuse her. She had her brain removed."

The surgery resulted in another, rather bizarre cognitive change. While the procedure sometimes caused spinal fluid to leak through the nose, in my case, the fluid just collected in the side of my head, creating a bulge.

Dr. Jackson was quick to correct me when I said I had a spinal fluid leak. "You do not have a leak because it's not leaving your body."

So instead of a leak, I guess I had a pool—a very tiny wading pool. I could feel the fluid passing out of my skull and pooling in my temple under the skin next to my ear. Sometimes it flowed back and forth. I could be in the middle of a conversation at work when all of a sudden I would feel the fluid moving out of my skull, spurring a momentary state of confusion as though I had just been bonked on the head. When the fluid scurried back into the skull, I felt a lightness. If I was talking when this happened, I would stop midsentence, silently acknowledge the change, and then pick up where I'd left off. Still, some fluid always got left behind, so I never felt quite "right."

As the months wore on, the fluid moved less and less often, and the pool shrank. Then one day, about nine months after the surgery as I was walking across campus with Leona, a Vanderbilt legal counsel, sssooooooop! *All* the fluid remaining in the pool was sucked inside with one full, final slurp. I immediately felt euphoric, energetic, and clearheaded for the first time since the surgery!

Leona and I came to a fork in the campus walkway. She took one path, and I took the other. As soon as her back was turned, I skipped down the path toward my office with a huge half grin on my face. I felt fabulous. For those nine months, I had forgotten what it felt like to experience the lightness of feeling "good."

As I began to reimmerse myself in social activities, my self-esteem took a hefty whacking. In face-to-face conversations I often wondered how distracting it was that my right eye did not blink, or that only half my brow would furrow to express shock or concern, or that only half my lip turned upward when I smiled. A gaggle of thirteen-year-old girls revealed the truth.

When Shea and I attended our first Mother-Daughter Book Club gathering since my surgery, the looks I got from some of the daughters would have sent even the most stoic of ugly ducklings crawling back to the nest. I walked into the meeting at Sarah and Lori's house and immediately gravitated to the sofa, and over the next hour, my eyes combed the circle of these young teens as each of them stole glimpses of Shea's Freak-Mother.

Horror, worry, pity—all were communicated in the first, second, and third glances. They couldn't get enough. Their attempts to hide their uncomfortable reactions were almost comical. It was hard to keep a straight face when I spoke. Shea was struggling as well. Thirteen is not the age you long for your parental units to demonstrate their individuality in public.

Thankfully, Shea integrated this and other flustering experiences into a mature perspective of her purpose and place in the world, an observation expressed by her teachers. Later, at the wise old age of twenty-five, Shea reported a litany of positive outcomes she experienced as a teen.

"While my friends were freaking out about the small stuff, I was able to blow much of it off....I was able to help my friends put the small things into perspective....I didn't take life for granted and was quick to help others see the positive side....I learned the importance of living a healthy life both physically and mentally, like dealing with whatever's bothering you so it doesn't take away from the rest of your life."

At the same time, Shea developed a fear of blood and needles along with a fear of losing her mother. Still, she and I are likeminded on this one—the constructive lessons far outweighed her fears.

By summer, six months into my new job, my battery was still not charged, but I was easing forward in a positive direction with a dribble here and a dollop there of extra stamina. With more energy, I took regular, snail-paced strolls down our mile-long driveway through the woods. As the gossamer greens of spring turned to the dense verdancy of summer, my senses delighted in the subtleties of Mother Nature's seasonal changes. I likened it to the magnified smells and sounds a blind person must experience. My frail hearing, balance, and cognition, combined with a dramatically buoyed spirit, created a keen awareness of the delicate movements, colors, and textures of the surrounding pasture and forest.

One hot, humid day in July, 1999, I toddled down the driveway admiring Mother Nature's 3-D canvas, as star-struck as a backwoodswoman on her virgin trip to New York City. The psychedelic indigo buntings were gliding frantically about, and the ovenbirds were whistling their repetitive tunes. As my eyes followed a frenzied tiger swallowtail butterfly diving up, down, and around for a smidgen of nectar, I spotted the blackberry thicket, laden with ripe berries. I was prepped for the battle, bucket in hand.

Blackberry picking can be a torturous endeavor, not suitable for the uninitiated. On that day, at that moment, with greatly heightened senses and a ravenous appetite for the joy of country living, I found my own little Garden of Eden. I reached into the mass of thorny branches and lightly tugged on the berries nestled among the leaves. The ripe berries dropped off one by one into my bucket. With each movement, thorns pierced my arms, and within fifteen minutes, my arms and hands were dotted with tiny freckles of blood, my shirt was soaked with sweat from the full sun and ninety-degree heat which blackberries adore, and the salty sweat was dripping in my eyes. The berries became fuzzy, dark-looking clumps.

Yet I was in Shangri-la. Working for these condensed little packets of energy seemed like the right thing to do. I paused in this maudlin state of mind to give a prayer of thanks: *Hold on to this feeling, Minda. Deposit securely into your memory bank the wince of the thorn's prick, the salty drips of sweat rolling into your eyes, and the confining second skin of drenched clothes—tactile symbols of being alive on a bountiful corner of the earth.*

Sweltering heat, stifling humidity, juxtaposed against the sweetness of the berries on my half-tongue—it was a worthy quest.

chapter fifteen

1999, SUMMER

In the summer of 1999, as my stamina tiptoed out of hibernation, my curiosity about ways to catalyze the healing process intensified. Barry and I attended the biennial symposium of the Acoustic Neuroma Association (ANA) in Milwaukee.

The ANA was founded by Fickel Ehr who was diagnosed in 1977 with a large acoustic neuroma. She had been alone in her layperson search for understanding the nature of the AN beast and the best treatment to rid herself of the tumor with the least damage. She could not find literature she understood, or first-person accounts from the patient's perspective. The surgery left her with significant neurological deficits and no support system, no one who understood the overwhelming effect of the treatment on her well-being. Due to this, she was inspired to make sure other AN victims did not have to repeat her experience.

At the time I attended the symposium, facial weakness still defined my appearance. When I entered the room with two hundred other struggling AN patients, I felt as if I'd come home. *My people—these are my people!*

With each workshop, I became more informed about what was broken and why, and how it could be mended. Health care experts from around the country opened door after door, confirming I was not a hypochondriac whose pity parties had gone over the top. My AN cronies and I walked out of each workshop plastered with our half smiles, gleeful we were not alone. The experience also obliterated any speck of doubt about my choice of treatment or surgeon.

Jackie Diels, an occupational therapist, led the most impressive workshop. She discussed retraining the brain to get the facial muscles moving in the right direction for the right emotion. Jackie's presentation started with a stunning photographic montage of celebrities whose emotionally charged faces we all knew—Michael Jordon, determined, but pained as he leaped for a ball; *Braveheart* warrior Mel Gibson, stoic in his fourteenth century Scottish uniform; a smiling President George Herbert Bush. No sound accompanied the montage. These familiar faces were gradually replaced with faces, faces and more faces—paralyzed and lacking expression.

Next on the screen were models displaying a range of facial expressions – grieving, joyful, quizzical. Eventually these fully functioning faces were juxtaposed with the contorted expressions of AN patients until the only images on the screen were their silly half snarls, half puckers and half moon smiles. One frame with eight words ended the slide show: *The face is the image of the soul.*

The contrast was striking—slapstick humor, Jim Carrey style. Another welcomed confirmation of a

misunderstood handicap. As Jackie launched into her talk
on repairing broken facial movements, I had to sit on my
hands to keep from leaping out of my seat with delight.

After the workshop, I cornered Jackie and said, "I
really enjoyed your workshop. I'd like to come see you
in Madison. I had a 2.2-centimeter tumor pushing on
the brain stem."

AN patients disclose the size of their tumors in the
same way recovering alcoholics proclaim their years of
sobriety. Jackie listened patiently while I talked.

"After the surgery, I had no movement at all, but a
little movement is coming back."

"I can definitely see some movement," she said. "I
also see some muscle cramping. Does your cheek hurt?"

"Does my cheek hurt?" I repeated the question
because I was unclear what she meant.

"Yes. Is your cheek sore?"

I tried to concentrate on how my cheek felt.

"Try this," she said. "Place your thumb inside your
mouth and up against your cheekbone like this." She
inserted her thumb in her mouth just under the
cheekbone. I did the same.

"Now place your fore and middle fingers, like this,
on top of your cheek." Once again, she demonstrated
with her own fingers and cheek. "Now press against
your thumb very firmly. Do you feel a thicker spot—
almost like a knot?"

"Yes, I do. I've never noticed it before."

"Hold your thumb and fingers against each other.
Press them together *hard*. It may hurt. But press and
hold until the pain goes away."

I followed her instructions. Within thirty seconds the muscle began to relax, and the knot and achiness in my cheek disappeared. "I can't believe that!" I exclaimed. "I've been walking around all this time with a cramp and didn't even know it! My face feels so relaxed!"

"You probably have other muscles contracting as well. But we'll work on that when you come to Wisconsin. The cheek will contract again. You know what to do now."

We talked a few minutes longer about my surgery and what it would take to get insurance approval. We agreed to speak later by phone.

"Thank you so much. I can't wait to come and see you." I gave my new comrade a hug and skipped to my next workshop.

The hearing loss workshop was equally revealing. At the beginning of the session, the speaker posed a question to her eager-to-learn participants. "How many of you have lost all or part of your hearing?"

Most of us raised our hands.

"Who is hearing disabled?" Only a smattering of the thirty-plus folks raised their hands.

"I'm here to let you know *all* of you who raised your hand the first time are hearing impaired and have a disability recognized by the federal government. There are rules and regulations that may apply to you, to get assistance for your hearing disability. So let me ask again. Who is hearing disabled?"

Hands went up all over the room. I was beginning to feel uneasy because her opening was suspiciously reminiscent of a Twelve Step therapy program. She might as well have said, "You've taken step one to help identify and access the resources available to you." My shoulders tensed up as I waited for her to rearrange the chairs into a circle and pressure each of us to tell our stories. *Oh, no.*

Fortunately, the workshop leader did not rearrange the chairs. Neither did she ask for a volunteer to stand up and share his story. Whew! Instead, she talked of hearing aids which employers, theaters, and other large venues were required by the 1990 Americans with Disabilities Act to provide if requested. She passed around one of the assisted listening devices so we could try it on for size. Once again, I was astonished to learn how ignorant I'd been about the degree of my impairment. The device translated the sporadically garbled words and phrases from the workshop leader's mouth into complete sentences I could fully understand. I departed the workshop with yet another hardy half-smirk.

Later in the day, a panel of surgeons validated my frustrations over my lack of energy. I learned extreme fatigue for weeks, months, and sometimes even longer was a universal symptom among AN surgical patients. The panel of experts debated the cause, never coming to any grand conclusion. I could not get up the guts in the audience of hundreds to raise my hand and give the patient's point of view: *Excuse me, Misters Smarty Pants, but you would be extremely fatigued, too, if your body was straining every minute of every day to hear, think, maintain your balance, move obstinate, cramped muscles in your face, block dry air and debris from blowing into your blink-impaired eye, and keep saliva and food from falling out of your mouth!*

Apparently, my long-held tendency to voice my opinions (loudly) was tossed out with my hearing. I sat quietly, comforted by an explanation for the fatigue that had suddenly congealed in my mind.

The panel also ruminated on plausible theories for the cognitive and memory loss reported by some AN surgical patients. Once again, they could not validate any scientific explanations, but they posed a rational theory. During surgery, the blood supply could be cut off or decreased to nearby parts of the brain, affecting other functions. At last, I had an excuse for my cognitive deficits.

Upon my return from the conference, one of my AN sisters sent me a silk-screen for a T-shirt. *Hello, my name is Minda. I've had a brain tumor. What is your excuse?* All in all, I got my money's worth of morale-boosting information and camaraderie from the symposium.

Back at home, I dove headfirst into the insurance quagmire to obtain approval for the facial retraining program with Jackie Diels. Hoops and health insurance coverage go together like a boo-boo and a Band-Aid. *You want to do what?*

It took only eight communications with my appropriately named Health 1.2.3 insurance provider. After appeals of two denials, they finally ceded to my pleas for mercy. Three months after learning of this newfangled way to coerce my face into cooperation, I was on the plane to Madison with my mother for an intensive three-day therapy program with Jackie at the University of Wisconsin Hospital and Clinics.

Day one with Jackie was half diagnostic, half educational, half massage—a very packed day. She broke the ice with the obligatory rapport-building conversation in which she allowed me to recite the full version of my saga. During this outpouring of my heartfelt recall, Jackie shrewdly began her evaluation of the facial damage. When I was done, she showed me a line drawing of a woman's face with the skin removed to expose the network of facial muscles. Helga, as Jackie called her, initially struck me as one of the Marvel Comics heroes whose disfigurement was the source of power. She had an angular, gripping kind of beauty with expressive eyes that elicited an immediate tinge of fondness.

"Notice all the muscles on Helga's face. The face and mouth take up more space on the movement control center of the brain than any other part of the body. The complexity of these small facial muscles gives humans the ability to communicate a wide range of emotions. In order to understand how this retraining program works, we're going to talk about the mechanics behind the varied facial expressions and what went wrong when you had the tumor removed."

"I love this stuff. Please go on."

"As you probably know, muscle movement is controlled by our nerves. Nerves are like cables. They're filled with a network of fibers extending the entire way from the brain to the muscle they're controlling."

As she talked, I bent closer to see the drawing better.

"The facial nerve alone contains six to seven thousand fibers," she said. "Yet the base of the facial nerve, with all its fibers, is not much bigger than a single string of thin spaghetti, and it gets even thinner as it branches out. I'm sure you've heard about the cranial nerves by now—the nerves that connect to the brain stem, including the facial and acoustic nerves."

"Unfortunately, I'm all too familiar with these guys," I replied. "Every day I'm reminded of my long-gone acoustic nerve and my beat-up facial nerve—not to mention the other cranial nerves that took a hit."

"Then you probably know when Dr. Jackson removed your acoustic neuroma, he also took out your acoustic nerve. To get both the tumor and the nerve out, he had to tug and pull on the neighboring facial nerve, fraying or bruising some of those fibers. Does this make sense so far?"

"Makes perfectly good sense. Dr. Jackson explained most of this to me."

"Good. Stop me if something doesn't make sense. Did he tell you that, in time, you could get most of the function back?"

"Yes, but he was honest with me—which I really liked. He said it was hard to tell how much movement I might regain. He said time would tell, but hopefully, most and maybe all of the movement would come back. He also said it might take time because nerves repair themselves very slowly, and he had to do quite a bit of wrestling with the facial nerve to get all of the little creep out."

"Yes. Nerves are very slow-growing, but eventually the swelling goes down, the frayed fibers grow back, and then the muscles start moving again. But herein lies the problem. Remember those thousands of fibers I mentioned?"

I nodded, not wanting to interrupt what was like a nail-biting bedtime story for me.

"You can imagine as the tiny, tiny fibers grow back, it can be quite a stretch, so to speak, for them to hook up at the same place they started before the surgery. Inevitably, some fibers grow back and connect up with the wrong guy."

"Like divorcees on the rebound," I said.

"Yes." She laughed. "Look in your mirror and smile."

I pulled out the small circular tabletop mirror Jackie had instructed me to bring. I set it on the table in front of me and assumed my serial killer grin—an especially uncomfortable assignment when your teacher is a couple of feet away scrutinizing your every move.

"What happens when you smile?" she asked.

"My smile looks silly. The right side of my mouth still doesn't go very far. I look like a doofus."

"Oh, I'm sure it doesn't look as good as before the surgery, but that's what we're here for. Smile again, and notice what happens to your right eye when you smile."

I looked in the mirror again. "It sort of winks when I smile." I looked like a deranged Mae West who couldn't turn off the urge to flirt.

"Exactly. Your smiling nerve fibers grew back and plugged into a port of the muscle that closes the eye. The brain is reading the old message. It doesn't know any better. This condition is called synkinesis."

"Synkinesis," I repeated.

Jackie nodded. "So you're going to retrain your brain to do the *right* thing when you smile. I'm going to teach you how to relax the circular eye muscle, and you're going to do that over and over again until the brain gets the point, and it becomes a habit. Eventually when you smile, it will automatically follow the new interpretation to stay open, rather than the old command to shut the eye."

"Wow. Sounds complicated," I said.

"Actually, the basics are simple but require a lot of concentration and patience. Teaching the nerves—or re-teaching them—is not quick and easy. We're going to take it a step at a time, so hopefully it will be easy enough to do. Before we get started, I want to take some photographs so we'll have the baseline documented and can gauge the progress you're making over time. I'll take photographs each time you come back."

"Cool."

Jackie took several shots of my face with her Polaroid, capturing a variety of expressions Diane Arbus style. Smile. Snarl. Surprise. The last time my face had been professionally photographed, my seventeen-year-old bare shoulders were framed in a pale pink fur stole, intended to help me look deserving of a high school diploma. As Jackie clicked away, I envisioned my modeling debut as a freak in a neurological publication.

Jackie gave me a big smile. "Let's move on to tackling those knots in your face."

Jackie said she saw several overly excited muscles contracted in place like a cramp. She explained that when those slow-growing nerve fibers finally did make it to their destination and connect up with the other side, they got overly excited and began to contract involuntarily. This excessive contraction was the reason electrical stimulation worsens the condition.

"Did anyone tell you to use electrical stimulation to help the muscles stay in shape until the nerves grow back?" she asked.

"Yes!" I said. "The physical therapist I saw after the surgery suggested it. Fortunately, Dr. Jackson forewarned me this treatment would exacerbate the problem, although if he told me why, it didn't sink in. So I told the PT thanks, but no thanks, and I never went back. I knew that woman didn't have a clue about what was going on in my face. The good news is when Health 1.2.3 asked why I couldn't go to a therapist here in Nashville instead of Wisconsin, I was able to paint a graphic picture of the problem."

"Good for you *and* Dr. Jackson for avoiding a common pitfall. Electrical stimulation is the exact opposite of what these muscles need. So now let's talk about a treatment we know works to relax those muscles—facial massage. We're going to work on three areas, your cheek, your chin, and the inside corner of your eyebrow."

Jackie started with the cheek and repeated the demonstration she had shown me in Milwaukee at the ANA Symposium. At the end of the exercise, my face felt as though a network of taut rubber bands had been released, relieving the year-old straightjacket of tension.

The next morning at eight o'clock, Jackie and I got down to work right away. I was her sole focus of attention for the entire day.

Retraining the brain is serious business. The brain is an obstinate prima donna who has to be told a command dozens of times before she finally submits. Objective Number One for gaining control of my titular princess was stopping her from ordering up a feeble wink when I smiled. Jackie explained how we were going to lasso Princess Brain into submission to do the right thing at the right time. We had four simple tools for taking charge, my tabletop $4.99 makeup mirror, the eight-by-ten drawing of Helga, my face, and my weary but seasoned meditation skills.

"I'm going to break this down into four steps. Just let me explain it to you first, and then you try it as I walk you through the steps. So just listen now.

"The first step is to relax your face—all the facial muscles as best you can. Step two is to make a tiny smile while you watch your eye in the mirror. Step three—freeze the smile as soon as you see your eye start to shut down.

"The fourth and final step is the tough one. While watching your eye in the mirror, hold the tiny isolated smile as you relax the muscles under your eye that are causing it to close. This step takes the greatest concentration. You want to actually feel the individual muscle contracting as you smile and then relax that same muscle as you hold the smile *and* relax the tightness under the eye.

"It's this muscle here you will focus on." She pointed to the eye muscle on Helga's face. "You will repeat these four steps at least three times each day. By doing this over and over again, you will lay down a new message in the brain that the eye should stay *open* when you smile, not begin to close. Eventually, the eye will act on its own like it used to." She paused to let all of this information sink in.

"What do you think? Ready to try it?"

"Yes. I think so."

"Okay. Let's give it a try. I'll talk you through it, step by step. So get your mirror ready."

I was a little nervous at this point. To get to this place, I had spent many hours chasing the approval of the insurance gods, then traveled about five hundred miles. It was all up to me now. I fiddled with the makeup mirror, placing it on top of a few books and adjusting the angle so it was closer to eye level. There staring back at me was Ms. Minda, cockeyed smile and all.

"Now keep staring into the mirror while you relax the muscles in each part of your face," Jackie said. "Start with your forehead, and keep the image of Helga's muscles in mind. Can you feel the tugging of the individual muscles?"

"Definitely. Amazing. Now that you've pointed it out, I can feel the muscles stretching to pull my eye closed."

"See how your left eye is opened wider than your right eye? See if you can relax the area around the right eye so the eye opens up more."

She observed my attempts. "That's it! See your eye opening up?"

"Yes. This is actually easier than I thought it was going to be."

"Now focus on relaxing the muscles in and around your cheek. Ooohhh. You did that quickly. Now focus on your chin. Ahhh. You've got it!"

"Yes, I could feel the tugging on both my chin and lower lip." I continued my attempt to keep the muscles relaxed. This relaxing was hard work.

"Okay. Let's move on to the next step. Keep gazing into the mirror with your face as relaxed as possible. Now smile a teeny, tiny smile—as small a smile as you can make."

As I looked into the mirror, I made my goofy smile.

"Nope. Too big. Go back to the relaxed state, and let's start again."

Uh-oh. I had been feeling pretty good about responding to her commands. All of a sudden, I felt the teacher was not happy with my performance.

"This time, as you very, *very* slowly turn the corners of your mouth up for a tiny, tiny smile, observe the movement of your right eye. As soon as you see your right eye start to close, stop, freezing both the smile and the squinted eye in place."

Sure enough, as I gazed at myself in the mirror and made an almost undetectable, sly little smirk, I watched my eye involuntarily start to close. I could feel the muscle being naughty.

"This is the synkinesis we talked about. Now relax, and let's do it again. But this time, make the tiny smile just big enough to see the eye start to close, and then hold it until I tell you what to do next."

I made the teeny smile, feeling my cheeks move upward on my face. As soon as the eye started to close, I stopped.

"Good. Feel the muscle tugging on the eye and forcing it to close?"

"Yep."

"Now, here comes the tricky part. Keep gazing at your right eye. Try and relax the muscle under the eye while holding the smile."

This last step was like rubbing your tummy while patting your head. I tried several times with no success. It required almost hypnotic, undivided attention. As soon as I relaxed the eye, my smile disappeared. The moment I smiled again, the eye mischievously squinted as if it had a mind of its own. I relaxed the eye, and the smile disappeared. This was not helping. I was confusing my brain, sending mixed messages. Smile. Squint. No, no, don't squint!

Finally, on try number five, just as I was losing hope, I held the smile and felt the eye muscle respond to my command. With my Mona Lisa smirk frozen in place, the muscle relaxed and my eye opened up!

"You've got it! Want to try again?"

"Yes!" I felt I had just solved Rubik's Cube, but with a practical purpose. "Boy, that last time around, I could feel the individual muscle pulling my eye closed, and then I could feel it relax as the eye opened. That is so cool!"

"It's remarkable, isn't it? Let's try it again."

I assumed the focused, mesmeric state again to tease out the *feel* of the individual muscles contracting. When the brain sent its inappropriate command to the eye, I took control and relaxed the tense muscle, opening my eye back up. It worked, an eye-opening experience!

"You did it again! You actually learned this pretty fast. It isn't an easy thing to do. Try it one more time."

The third time was more of a challenge. I struggled to get my eye muscle to relax while my smile was on hold. I could feel the tug, but could not deliver the command to make it relax. I was under pressure. Pressuring myself to relax didn't work. *Focus, Minda. Be Here. Be Now. Feel the muscle.* Bingo! I pulled it off again. I was in command.

"All right. Good job. I want you to write down the steps, so when you get home tonight, you can try it again. It may be harder tonight. Most people find when they're tired, it's harder to do. After a few days, you can make a little bit bigger smile—just a tiny bit bigger— and then once you've mastered that, a bigger smile, until the eye stays open automatically."

By the end of the three-day visit, I was loaded down with massages, a heating pad, and three sets of movement patterns for the eye closure and lop-sided snarl.

Our final day in Wisconsin was spent touring the rural countryside. Snow fell on the late October day when Mom and I drove to Taliesin, Frank Lloyd Wright's infamous home on the outskirts of Madison. I left Wisconsin with all the cockles of my heart and face aglow, savoring the greatly improved welfare of my facial present and future.

Back in Nashville, my undisciplined persona managed to stay with the program of repetitious repetitions. Staring at your face several times a day actually is quite fascinating. My eyes were like macro lenses focused for a close-up. I became intimate with every freckle, every crease, every pockmark on my weathered face. I developed X-ray vision that could "see" the facial muscles through the skin.

The retraining exercises got easier and easier, and the improvement was astonishing. I mastered the de-winking and stopped my involuntary eye closure. The benefit of a winkless smile was physically therapeutic as well as cosmetic. As the cramping and tugging became less frequent and the muscles relaxed, so did the rest of my body. Such focus on the face was as much a distraction from my numerous other ailments as fixing the door handle of our ramshackle '68 Chevy truck.

Over the next year, I made two more trips to Madison. By the final trip, my brain was as submissive as an obedient dog. My facial muscles sat when I told them to sit, and Dr. Jackson was so impressed, he requested Jackie's phone number for another patient.

During the last trip to Madison, Jackie gave me a set of movement patterns to guide me to my final destination—an even smile. Though I had greatly benefited from the exercises, I eventually ran out of steam and could no longer discipline myself to concentrate on tiny little facial muscles. So I never achieved the perfect smile.

As this low-achieving high achiever attempted to claw her way back into a routine schedule, I continued to feel a severely hampered energy reserve. When I lamented about the intensity of my fatigue to Dr. Jackson, he forewarned me some patients found it took three years to regain their energy. And sure enough, my body took that timetable to heart, finally attaining a reasonably adequate level of energy by the end of year three.

Whether it was just Surgery Number Eight or the synergistic effect of all the surgeries and other treatments combined, my rainy day reserve has never been totally replenished, even as I write this. A boxer can take a beating only so many times. He may win the tenth fight of his life, but halfway through fight eleven, his exhaustion may be beyond what the ding of a bell and a sixty-second break can assuage.

I can walk (usually in a straight line, but not always), talk (mostly coherently, but not always), and think (often disjointedly, but not always). Yet if I get tired or contract even the most innocuous virus, I'm a zombie. My face reverts to the weakness and synkinesis of the pre-Jackie era, and coherent thinking and speech slow to a snail's pace.

Barry has been the witness of the composite effect of my impediments. He has shown an incredible tolerance—mostly, but not always. Most of the time, Barry gives me strong encouragement to get off my ass, spiff myself up, and venture into the masses. More times than not, I receive a fresh dose of embarrassment when I encounter someone I haven't seen in a while. When I catch her up on my most recent escapades, her reply makes me cringe.

"Wow, you don't look so bad. I can hardly tell!"

Folks should remember, bad is not good when describing a woman's appearance.

As the years have rolled on, I've made other accommodations to the handicaps. Most of these adjustments have actually improved the quality of my life. For example, instead of meaningless small talk, cocktail parties now lead to intimate discussions with friends and colleagues. Here's how the scenario usually unfolds.

I sit at the quietest edge of the room and wait for a long lost friend to spot me. When she sees me, she raises her eyebrows in surprise as if to say, "I didn't know you were still alive!" Then she smiles. I point to the chair next to me, and she meanders over. Without the distraction of a five-way conversation, our dialogue is elevated above the superficial. Before you know it, we've made a meaningful connection, memorable enough to last until we see each other at the next party.

If I'm so unfortunate as to land in a five-way conversation, I hear only noise, and I am humbled either by my dumb silence or the inane responses I feel obliged to give. Sometimes I just stay home and read a good book—my favorite thing to do anyway.

2001

After the first ANA conference, I kept my eyes and ear open to learning more about the AN surgery and its side effects. Then in 2001, I attended another ANA Symposium. An in-depth conversation with a surgeon led to an eye-opening revelation. During a roundtable discussion, I asked him directly, "What is the single most important factor in minimizing damage to the surrounding nerves?"

He responded, "Encapsulation."

He explained that, when a tumor is confined to a specific area, surrounded by a thin layer of tissue, it is "encapsulated," and therefore much easier to remove. He told the following story to illustrate his point.

A patient with a very large acoustic neuroma, about the size of a golf ball, had emotionally prepared for a very long surgery. But when the surgeon got inside, the tumor was totally encapsulated, so it lifted off and away from the other nerves with relative ease. The surgery lasted only seven hours, and the patient suffered minimal facial damage. She and her family called the surgeon a hero. But the reality was the tumor's encapsulation had made the difference. If the tumor had been half that size, but not encapsulated, it would have taken longer and caused much greater damage to the surrounding nerves.

Dr. Jackson's "good guy, bad guy" reference now made all the more sense to me. The fact that he referred to my tumor as "a sticky, bloody mess that was not encapsulated" made my heart swoon for him. Dr. Jackson had never complained. He had never revealed the extent of the challenge he encountered in picking the tumor off my brain stem and saving the functions of my tongue, lips, throat, eye, smile, and cheek, not to mention my breathing and heartbeat. Thank you a million times over, Dr. Jackson, for sparing me and my cranial nerves.

By year four of the post-AN surgery saga, I was well on my way to an admirable quality of life with a balanced routine of working, mothering, wifing, homemaking, and volunteering—you know the routine working women carry these days. I buffered life's duties with plenty of sleep and limited exposure to uncontrolled sources of stress. With a family-and-wellness-friendly boss, and a thoroughly empathetic husband and daughter, I learned to say no.

No, sorry, wish I could help, but I just can't.

No. That sounds like a wonderful opportunity, but I have to say no.

No. Years ago I would have said an immediate yes, but these days, I unfortunately don't have the stamina. I hope you'll forgive me.

No.

The hard-earned lesson of repeatedly voicing the most underrated word in our vernacular afforded me the time and energy to be a devoted mother to my teenager and a faithful daughter to my aging parents. Parenting a teen rivals the stress of dealing with uncontrollable tumors. In fact, it may be even tougher. The task was lightened by my emotional availability. I still made my share of mistakes in guiding the grounded and rebelliously healthy Shea, but managed to keep my eyes focused and ear perked for the teen traps, regardless of my weariness.

2003

In late summer of 2003, we parted ways with our miracle child as she began her dual four-year stints as studious cowgirl and party animal at the University of Texas in Austin. Not long after arriving home from our drive halfway across the country and back, I had the bittersweet job of holding my father's hand as he passed from this life.

Despite years of contemplation about death, those final three weeks of holding, loving and learning from my father gave me an incomparably profound experience. It seemed both appalling and pre-ordained to learn so much in such a short time from the waning days of someone else's life. Yet observing a man confronting the end of life revealed secrets which seemed to be intended not just for him, but for the living as well.

In truth, it was not only my love that allowed me to be so present during the excruciating event, but also my mastery of saying *no. No, I cannot do anything else but be at my father's bedside.* With that singular focus, I opened myself up not only for a painful rite of passage but also for indelible lessons on the meaning and mindfulness of life. Surprisingly, those preternatural days by my father's bedside eased my return to an empty-nested family, my professional work, and ongoing healing.

2005

By 2005, almost eight years after the AN surgery, I felt comfortable with the plateau I had reached, more aware of both my limitations and my capabilities than I had ever been. I knew how to walk the tightrope of my Type-A activist persona and my type C physical capabilities. This balance had allowed me to maintain an excellent state of health for eight long years.

So when the Reach to Recovery volunteer called to ask me to speak at the luncheon, it was easy for me to say no.

She would not accept no, however. So a couple of months later, I found myself standing on the stage before a banquet hall of breast cancer survivors.

The speech was electrifying for me. The response from the audience was unexpected and overwhelming. After my speech as the crowd cleared out, the light bulb flashed in my head. I thought, *A book. It is time for me to write a book.*

Just as I was walking out of the room floating on my inflated ego, the floor seemed to open up like a sinkhole. I tilted off-balance, as if I were about to fall into the abyss. A moment later, the floor closed up and I regained my balance without falling.

Whoa, I must have pushed myself too hard, I thought. *Just the stress of the speech,* I rationalized.

Before I had a chance to give the book more thought, the balance problems became more frequent, although they were much more subtle than the illusion of a sinkhole. Other symptoms arose that were suspiciously similar to the acoustic neuroma symptoms I'd experienced eight years earlier, including lightheadedness, ringing in my good ear, and once again, a twitching eyelid. I also had vision trouble, with a loss of peripheral vision and a general worsening of both near- and far-sightedness. When the worry meter spiked too high, I made an appointment with Dr. Jackson.

After going through another MRI of the brain, Xanax would have been a handy accompaniment for my stroll from the hospital Imaging Department to Dr. Jackson's office. I kept telling myself, *Total deafness is not as bad as blindness.* I did my best to prepare for the worst, but it had taken me eight years to get where I was (where was I?).

Dr. Jackson walked into the examining room, and after our genteel salutations to bridge the gap of a four-year hiatus, he immediately got to the point. "I don't see any evidence of an acoustic neuroma. The imbalance most likely is the result of just getting older."

That's good news? I'm just getting older?

"Years ago after the surgery, your left balance nerve compensated for the loss of the nerve on your right side. But aging can cause a progressive *de-*compensation. A physical therapist can help you with that. For now, more importantly, you need to deal with something else first."

Something else? My good ear perked up.

He said, "There appears to be another growth on the MRI. Looks like in your jaw, maybe a schwannoma. The man you need to see is Dr. N. at Vanderbilt."

Dr. Jackson wisely chose not to elaborate, although he managed to diffuse my fear by assuring me it was probably benign. Even though I had a new tumor, I felt relieved. With the anxiety of another acoustic neuroma extinguished, the prison doors flew wide open, and I ran out as fast as I could. My heart and mind were already celebrating. No acoustic neuroma! No total deafness! No devastating fatigue! A jaw tumor? Shucks. I can handle that.

A follow-up appointment with Dr. N. revealed a small, most likely benign tumor, so we agreed to just wait and watch.

Five months later, I took the leap and resigned from MIHOW to give my body a break and settle down to write the book. I knew it was unrealistic to envision a level of stamina that would allow me to work full-time *and* complete a book. So in March, 2006, I turned in my resignation with sadness about leaving an exceptional program that attracted remarkable women to its rolls, but joyful with the excitement of devoting a year (or so I thought) to telling my story.

A few days after I announced my resignation to be effective in July, I was diagnosed with another brain tumor.

chapter sixteen

2006, MARCH

March 30, 2006. I was perched on the edge of the examining table poised for Dr. N.'s arrival. Dr. N. and I were to discuss when he would escort the benign jaw tumor to the hinterlands. Since the growth was wedged in the recesses of my neck at the back of my jaw, there was no need for disrobing. I sat fully clothed, staring at the closed, drab clinic room door. The door opened, but instead of Dr. N., it was the Vandy resident-of-the-semester. I had met this young man a few minutes earlier when he performed the perfunctory "I'm here to learn" check-in.

His flat, awkward countenance displaced the cheerful smile from our earlier encounter. He was making an obvious attempt to mask some other emotion—concern perhaps? As he sat down on the stool next to me, he opened my folder and stared at the page a moment, then turned to me. My eyes wandered to the open record. The word *meningioma* jumped off the page. It was one ten-letter word amidst dozens of others, but it instantly filled the center of my vision. It might as well have been highlighted in twenty-point type. It was the only word I saw.

Meningioma.

I was ignorant of its meaning, but I intuitively knew it was ominous. Neither Dr. Jackson nor Dr. N. had mentioned the word to me when I was last seen six months earlier.

"Partialities often make people see more than exists," Mark Twain once mused.

In those few seconds between the resident opening the file and preparing to speak, my mind had conjured up a cantankerous brain tumor in flashing browns and reds already eating away at my future.

Before I had a chance to wander farther down this path of imaginary horrors, the resident said, "Dr. N. will be here in a minute. We see something else on your MRI, another tumor . . ." Pause.

"What is it?"

"I'll let Dr. N. tell you about it. He knows much more than I do and will explain it more clearly."

At that moment, Dr. N. walked in. "Hello! Good to see you again! How are you?"

Dr. N., the crème de la crème of neck surgeons in Nashville, had a personable bedside manner, reminding me of a jolly, slimmer version of the Pillsbury Doughboy. His effusive friendliness had the immediate effect of displacing the tension with a lighter, convivial mood, softening the thud of bad news.

"I *was* doing well. But I'm not sure now. You tell me."

"It doesn't look like the tumor in your jaw has changed much. Good news. But we see something else on your MRI, though. Looks like a meningioma. These tumors are almost always benign growths in the lining, or meninges, of the brain."

Within a millisecond, my brain was back in that nebulous place of no thought. A leaden numbness encased a fiery concoction of fear and déjà vu.

Dr. N. continued, "This tumor is outside my territory. I'm a neck guy, from here down." He pointed to the back of his jaw down to the throat. "The priority right now is to determine the appropriate treatment for this tumor. You may need surgery, or maybe radiation is the best treatment."

I had the presence of mind to say, "I'm fairly certain I won't be able to have any more radiation. We already visited that option with the acoustic neuroma, and I was told I had received more than my fair share of radiation when I was treated for the Hodgkin's."

"Well, if surgery is the best option, we may be able to remove both the meningioma and the mandibular lesion at the same time."

"You mean I could get a two-for-one bargain?"

He smiled. "Again, this is not my area of expertise. You'll need to talk with a neurosurgeon to help you make that decision. There are two fine surgeons in town. You probably want to see Dr. H. who does surgery with Dr. Jackson. Or if you want to stay here at Vanderbilt, Dr. Reid Thompson is a terrific surgeon also."

The rest of the consultation with Dr. N. was brief. Before we parted ways, he leaned forward to grab my hand, looked me in the eye from just inches away, and said, "I'm sorry."

At least that's what I think he said. He was closer to my deaf ear, so the words may have been a bit jumbled.

Still, I found those two words both comforting and alarming.

As soon as I got out of the hospital, I released all the emotion held back over the previous half hour via a downpour of tears and heavy breathing. With the top off the pressure cooker, I called Barry.

"I just left Dr. N.'s office. The tumor in my jaw hasn't grown much, if at all, but I have another problem."

"Now what?"

"I have some kind of growth in my brain. He says it looks like a benign tumor." With the audible sounds of *brain* and *tumor*, I spilled the contents of my one serviceable tear duct again.

"Oh, Minda. Not again."

"He's referred me to two brain surgeons. We'll talk about it when I get home. I'm walking to the car and will be home soon."

I ended the call abruptly. I didn't want to talk about it. It was time to wallow in the numbness—to store up energy for the research for my next tumor thesis. My bookshelf at home was already sagging from the weight of prior investigations, but the shelf's ability to accommodate endless reams of information seemed to be one of those magical feats of technology, like the magnetic relationship between my gut and Jell-O— there's always room for more.

Dear Reader who has hung in there for fifteen chapters of spoiled body parts, are you exhausted by hearing of the Misadventures of Minda's Fertile Tumor Gardens? We are in the home stretch. Here's the streamlined, four-part tale of the next major surgery, Surgery Number Nine in case you've lost count: The

Research, Getting Psyched, The Surgery, and The Aftermath.

Phase I: The Research

I began my research with a few simple, but significant tidbits of information: the names of two brain surgeons and the probable type and location of the tumor—a meningioma in the optic chiasm. The two surgeons were Dr. H., who'd been part of the Olympic team for my eight-hour acoustic neuroma surgery, and Dr. Reid Thompson of Vanderbilt. I knew no practical details about either guy. I knew absolutely nothing about meninges or the optic chiasm, though the latter sounded breathtaking.

The next day, my computer and I went on a little journey. We surfed until we uncovered a Web site noting in graphic detail the various locations of meningiomas and their respective likelihood of cancer. I learned the optic chiasm is a meeting place where the two nerves controlling sight for each of the eyes form a juncture. Tumors in the meninges of the optic chiasm, as well as in any of the meninges of the brain, are almost always benign.

With an elementary understanding of the intruder's home base, I was ready to meet with the two potential directors of this additional act to my seemingly never-ending play. My hopes and energy were charged for the task ahead. Another success was in my future.

Consultations with Drs. H. and Thompson, and additional queries by phone with their colleagues, revealed the following data. Only one person in Nashville, other than Dr. N., had heard of Dr. Thompson because he was relatively new in the crowd of Vanderbilt doctors. He had moved to Nashville from LA where he had practiced at the famous Cedars-Sinai Medical Center. He was young enough to have very steady hands, but old enough to convey confidence in his experience. His estimation for the time of the job from start to finish was around six to seven hours. Dr. Thompson was as amiable and easy to converse with as your favorite professor.

Dr. H. also was a very unassuming, likable guy with hundreds of hours of flight time. His fingers were a bit bulkier than Dr. Thompson's, a detail that caught Barry's eye. He estimated the surgery would take three to four hours. The word on the street regarding Dr. H. came from several physicians, but the most important perspective was from someone who had worked side-by-side with him in the OR, Dr. Jackson.

"He's a road warrior—an excellent surgeon. I would strongly recommend him."

Dr. Jackson admitted he had not heard of Dr. Thompson, "who may very well be a good surgeon," but encouraged me to consider the "road warrior." I interpreted this to mean that the man doing surgeries day after day might be preferable to a surgeon who devoted many hours to research and teaching.

This first shot at fact gathering did not summon a clear sign about which guy to cast as director, so I lollygagged in noncommittal while I carried on with my research. The next steps were a face-to-face consultation with Dr. H. and a little more digging on the reputation of the new kid on the block, Dr. Thompson.

Ten days after my diagnosis, my research came to an abrupt halt. The day began with a meeting with Potential Brain Surgeon Number Two, Dr. H., for "the interview." During the discussion, I mentioned the option of seeking an opinion from St. Jude about how to handle the jaw tumor in light of the discovery of the meningioma. Dr. H. sent us over to a diagnostic center to pick up a copy of the MRI to send to St. Jude. We were in the center's lobby, waiting for the disk, when Barry's cell phone rang.

Barry left the building and took the call outside the clinic door. It was Robbie, his sister's husband. His mother Chickie had checked into the hospital in Memphis on Saturday after collapsing on a short walk. They were running tests to determine what was wrong. Robbie hesitated getting to the point. Even though he was a neurologist with twenty-three years' experience, spilling the news of his mother-in-law's death must have been excruciating.

"They were running a test on Chickie this morning when she had another event . . . and she died."

Chickie, this formerly healthy-as-an-ox, eighty-two-year-old woman, died just forty-five days after her beloved Norm died. In the span of seven weeks, Barry had lost both his mother and father, and his wife was diagnosed with another brain tumor. What was next?

We buried Chickie two days later. Although our grieving would last for months (it seemed like years) for loss of mother, father, mother-in-law, father-in-law, grandfather, grandmother, on April 13, three days after her sudden death, we began to mop up the emotional mess to clear room in our psyches for making decisions. It was time to choose when and how someone was going to reach inside my skull once again and yank out the newest interloper.

Serendipitously, the Memphis funeral was convenient for a visit to St. Jude Hospital for a second opinion about my jaw tumor. The so-called meningioma, by virtue of its location, had sucked up all my attention, but her cousin in my jaw was also still ruffling the remaining fragments of my peace of mind.

A couple of hours with the St. Jude doctors led to a workable solution. They were of the same opinion as Dr. N. The jaw tumor had all the features of a noncancerous growth, so there was no reason to rush into removing it at the same time of the meningioma surgery. Dr. Hudson recommended a needle biopsy, however, to ease my mind. A tangible sign of benign cells would let my nagging worry meter settle down. Although there was no urgency, because of my history she suggested the jaw tumor be removed after I healed from the brain surgery.

Back in Nashville after the funeral, the needle biopsy was quickly scheduled. This simple procedure provided no conclusive results, but the absence of a definitive diagnosis of cancer helped me shift my focus.

With Dr. Jackson's unequivocal vote of confidence, I was leaning toward Dr. H., yet Barry was leaning toward Dr. Thompson for obscure reasons. Dr. Thompson was younger and reminded him of a professional athlete in the prime of his career. It seemed clear we would be in good hands with either surgeon. So I called Uncle Stanley in LA to see if he could tap into the Cedars-Sinai doctor party line for the local scuttlebutt on Dr. Thompson's tenure. Uncle Stanley called back two days later with the inside scoop.

"I talked with a former colleague who worked with Dr. Thompson at Cedars-Sinai, and he said he was such a terrific surgeon they had begged him to stay. He's the kind of surgeon who carefully plans in advance the steps he'll take for each possible scenario. He told me this guy is as good as it gets, and with absolutely no reservations he would choose him to be the surgeon for himself or his family. You would be in the best of hands."

"Thank you, thank you, thank you, Uncle Stanley. You have made my day! This is the news I was waiting to hear—an opinion from someone who has stood side-by-side and observed him in action."

With the background data on Dr. Thompson now filled, plus the knowledge that surgery at Vandy could be cheaper because of my Vanderbilt employee insurance, I was beginning to lean toward Dr. Thompson. One additional bit of information would complete the puzzle: Why did Dr. Thompson estimate six to seven hours while Dr. H. said three to four hours?

I called my friend Dr. Jeanne Ballinger who had performed both of my mastectomies. I could rely on her unquestionable ethics and her sincere devotion to help patients make informed decisions.

"My guess is that both of them are giving their best estimates," she said, "but one is erring on the short side, and the other is erring on the long side. Dr. H. may be focusing on the primary surgical time from the opening to the closing of the skull, while Dr. Thompson may have included all the time from when you are taken to OR to when you are rolled into the recovery room."

"What about the fact that Vandy is a teaching hospital? Do you think that makes any difference?"

"It may make a little difference, but probably not much. I know Dr. H. is a fine surgeon. I don't know Dr. Thompson since I've been out of the Vanderbilt loop for a while, but I do know Vanderbilt has been recruiting the best surgeons from around the country. I believe both surgeons will use whatever time it takes to do the best job they possibly can."

With this final piece of the puzzle, we cast our chips with Dr. Thompson.

Meanwhile, both Drs. Thompson and H. had strongly encouraged me to get a baseline assessment of my vision damage to provide a measure of the surgery's success. Before the diagnosis, I had attributed my inability to read maps to the usual fifty-one-year-old's expiring warranty on eyesight. The diagnosis of the meningioma in the optic chiasm indicated a more sinister cause of the loss of vision.

The ophthalmologist, Dr. M., had treated me several years earlier for tear duct and eye closure problems stemming from the acoustic neuroma surgery. Because she was a Vandy physician with a superlative reputation, medical students and residents were following her around, nipping at her heels to observe her examination of my eyes.

When it was over, I asked, "May I talk with you in private, please?" That is, *I'd like to get your totally honest response, not colored for the benefit of your disciples.*

After the students left the room, I explained my dilemma of choosing between these two physicians. At first, Dr. M. replied as the other physicians did, "They are both very good surgeons with excellent reputations. You probably can't go wrong with either. I've not been in a surgery with Dr. H., but I have been in a couple of surgeries with Dr. Thompson, and he is one of the best surgeons I've seen in action. In fact, he is one of the two best surgeons I've ever worked with, anywhere."

She went on to explain, "A lot of the success depends on the tumor, for instance, where it's located. Let me take a look at your MRI."

She left the room and came back in a couple of minutes. She sat down on the stool, looked at my open chart on the table, then turned to me and said, "There is a huge risk of the lights going out."

"What did you say?" I wanted to make sure I had heard her *incorrectly*.

"There is a *huge* risk the lights will go out." Period. No convoluted message veiled with enigmatic medical jargon.

I resisted fully comprehending her warning. "What do you mean?" I was reaching for a simple explanation I might have missed.

"Your tumor is sitting in the optic chiasm where the nerves controlling your vision come together. Sometimes these tumors share a blood supply with these nerves, so even though the surgeon may preserve the optic nerves, they will no longer function if the blood supply is cut off."

Her facial expression matched her words—a look of very serious concern.

"Wow. Thank you for telling me this. Your opinion, your direct explanation of what you see, is what I need to hear, although it's quite shocking."

Whisssh. Back into that numbing, inert space. I truly appreciated her directness. I had asked for it. Now what should I do with the information? I shackled my emotions long enough to get the hell out of Dodge. On the walk back across campus toward my office, I called Barry. His response was once again the calm voice of reason.

"Call Dr. Thompson. See what he has to say about this. Something is missing. Neither surgeon mentioned this."

As soon as I got to the office, I called Tracy, Dr. Thompson's nurse.

"He's out of town, but I'm sure he would have mentioned this to you if he thought it was a problem. He's really good about that," she said convincingly.

I made another appointment with Dr. Thompson to get clarification about the range of risks and his experience in this part of the brain. I felt compelled to look him in the eye and imprint in my memory a detailed image of his capabilities to stop the dribbles of self-doubting. The mind never seems to shut up.

"There is always a risk," Dr. Thompson told me later when I asked about the "huge risk of the lights going out." I did not tell him who told me this, as I did not want the source to hesitate to reveal valuable information to her other patients.

"This is my area of expertise," he said, "performing surgery around blood vessels, so I feel confident we can do this, though I can't guarantee anything."

We chatted a while, and I watched his hands. They were very steady. He was reassuring without being arrogant, defensive, or patronizing. He pledged that he and only he would perform the surgery, an essential confirmation to obtain when a difficult surgery is performed at a teaching hospital.

We then discussed the when and how. Delaying the surgery for two or three weeks until after Shea came home from college was reasonable, but not as long as a couple of months. We talked at length about how he was going to get in and out of my head—a major piece of the puzzle for me in order to clear the buzzing bees from my active mind.

Drill bits, screws, and titanium plates would be involved. With my head stabilized by a 'head holder,' the scalp and underlying muscle from my left forehead and temple would be cut and pulled forward and out of the way. The skull would be penetrated by two holes made with a high speed drill bit. Next the dura (leathery brain encasing) would be flayed, followed by a little more drilling through bone and skull. With microscopic equipment inserted through the holes of the skull, Dr. Thompson would then be able to reach in and lift the frontal lobe to get a bird's-eye view of the tumor and the optic nerves.

After separation of the tumor from the nerves, blood vessels, and other surrounding tissues, the skull would be put back together with two sets of titanium plates and screws. Dr. Thompson and his crew were master metal-workers, so the junctures would be seamless, with all construction debris swept away. No need to worry my hard little head. (Some of these details were obtained later from the post-operative report.)

Believe it or not, I floated out of the consultation with Dr. Thompson, feeling like I had just secured the Oscar of optic chiasm meningioma surgeries. My mind was liberated from questions about when, how, and by whom. I could now move on to getting in the most positive, relaxed frame of mind to help me prepare me for both the expected and the unforeseen.

Phase II: Getting Psyched

Twelve days before the surgery, I accompanied Barry to New Hampshire for an environmental conference at the historic 1902 Mount Washington Hotel, site of the 1944 Bretton Woods International Monetary Conference. We checked in at the historic front desk, were given our historic brass keys, and made our way up the two flights of stairs to our historic room. A bronze plaque was nailed to the door: *President and Mrs. George H. W. Bush.*

When Barry opened the door to our suite, complete with a party size living room and hot tub (not historic), and the panoramic view of the White Mountains, Barry puffed up his chest like he was President Bush himself. He assumed he had been given the room designated for the best of the invited speakers. Unbeknownst to him, we were being treated to this suite because he was a surprise honoree for a River Hero Award. Of course having a poor, pitiful wife with a brain tumor didn't hurt.

While Barry attended the conference workshops, I resumed a rigorous schedule of healing: meditate, massage, dine, hike, rest, swim (in the historic indoor pool), dine, read, rest, and dine again. Rest overnight and repeat.

I used the opportunity of unstructured time to play a little game in preparation for the worst. Schooling myself in the worst possible outcomes always eased the jitters about my future. I envisioned being visionless while performing rote tasks such as dressing, brushing my teeth, and eating. I tried navigating the stairs with my eyes closed. I got out of bed and made my way to the bathroom "blind." I found my tennis shoes, slipped them on my feet, and tied up the laces with eyelids shut tight—no cheating. Reading was another story. Life without reading was something I could not play around with.

As I simulated life without vision, I told myself the "blindzies" were not so bad. All in all, my try-outs for the role of a half-baked Helen Keller diffused the fear of a not-so-good ending. Later I learned Barry also was fighting off fears of a life with the blind model of Minda. He was scared we would not be able to cope.

As I wandered around the Mount Washington Hotel, I enjoyed telling strangers I was on a medical mission. It's not often you get to tell someone, "I have a brain tumor."

"Nice to meet you. No, I'm not a river activist. I'm not even a professional environmentalist. I have a brain tumor and came along for the ride to take advantage of the healing environment."

When I broke the news of my predicament, most people wanted to hear more, and I wanted to tell them more. I no sooner had begun the truncated version of my saga when I learned about someone's cousin who had a brain tumor, but was doing nicely. Or someone's sister who had breast cancer. Or a father who suffered from emphysema. All of these conversations were better than talking about Total Maximum Daily Loads of river pollution with these committed, one-tracked environmental professionals.

On the fourth and final evening of our stay, a banquet was held to honor environmental heroes around the country who had done a yeoman's job of saving a part of our fragile waterways. A few minutes before Barry's name was to be announced in front of this audience of two hundred, Barry leaned over to me and whispered, "I'm going to the bathroom."

He disappeared before I had a chance to stop him. After about five minutes, the co-conspirators of the surprise sent a friend to find him. The friend returned with Barry, and they quietly took their seats just in the nick of time. John, our friend and Barry's colleague, took the stage and gave an introduction of the unnamed awardee. When he finally disclosed the surprise River Hero's name, a photo of a thirteen-year-old Barry flashed on the big screen, fully adorned in Eagle Scout regalia, badges, hat, and all.

Barry was caught off guard—and delighted. The award solved the puzzler he had pondered for the past few weeks: *Why was Minda agreeing to this trip right before her surgery when she usually insisted on hunkering down and sliding into the OR fully relaxed?* Mystery solved.

By the time we returned to Nashville, I had one more week to go before The Day. In this final week, I was wined and dined by friends and family. With two days to go, a group of dear friends and neighbors threw me a bon voyage party at Tom and Brenda's homestead. The centerpiece of the event, other than the profuse love and well-wishing, was a display of cheeses from around the world adorned with little flags noting their places of origin. The evening was truly a gift, a group love fest that stayed with me all the way into the operating room.

The night before the surgery, we held the usual Last Supper with my varsity cheerleaders, Mom, Barry, Shea, and Ava. More love. I was one lucky gal. Still, I missed my deceased father's sweet farewell kiss planted on my cheek before each of my surgeries. He had disguised a lifetime of arthritic pain with his ever-durable sense of humor and dignity. His embrace had always helped give me the strength to keep my head and spirits high.

As Barry and I lay in bed that final night, I turned to him and said, "Oh! There is one really, really important thing I need to show you before tomorrow."

"What is it?" he asked, expecting the worst.

"You need to learn how to put on my makeup." I was still holding on to the vision of a reasonably good-looking deaf, dumb, and blind girl.

Phase III: The Surgery

At 4:30 a.m. on The Day, Barry, Shea and I arose, stumbled into our Prius half asleep, and drove to the Vandy Medical Center campus. At the entrance of the hospital, we paused for a photograph. Much like the image captured on the first day of a cruise, the three of us stood beside the Vanderbilt Hospital sign, memorializing our departure for this big adventure. I did not feel sick. In fact, I felt so good, it seemed like I was checking in for elective surgery. *I'd like to change my appointment to next Thursday, please.*

Within an hour, Barry and I were in the pre-op room, and I was sitting up on a gurney in a hospital gown, lightly covered with a sheet. A curtain surrounded the six-by-ten holding pod. I peered down at the IV which had just been inserted into my least favorite place, my hand. The resident anesthesiologist slipped inside my curtained altar.

"Hello. I'm from the Anesthesia Department, and I'll be assisting with your anesthesia. You must have connections. You've got the head of the our Department scheduled for your surgery."

"Yep. This is not my first time around. I guess they have mercy on me."

"Well, you're also in good hands with Dr. Thompson. He's the best. Any questions for me?"

"I just want to get the show on the road. I'd like a little feel good juice, though—you know, like the old days. Can you give me something that makes me smile from cheek to cheek, the stuff that lasts for a few minutes rather than immediately knocking me out?"

"Sure. No problem. The nurse will be here shortly." He left.

I felt quite calm and ready to roll. The curtain surrounding my gurney was pulled aside again, and in walked Dr. Thompson with his protégés.

"Well, I see you've been checking up on me. I got an e-mail from a former colleague. He said you were trying to find out how good a surgeon I am." Dr. Thompson had a sweet smile on his face.

"I guess I did do some checking around. That's my job. My uncle's a retired anesthesiologist in LA, and I asked him to check you out. Needless to say, I found out what I needed to know, and here we are! I was told I couldn't find a better surgeon than you. Are you ready to go?"

"Yes. I just had a long look at your MRI."

In that moment, on that gurney, with abundant faith in Dr. Thompson, and with a stillness in my soul, I was at peace and as ready as I could be for whatever lay ahead. "I'm ready, Dr. Thompson. Let's do it."

"All right. See you when you wake up." He slipped behind the curtains trailed by his wannabes.

I was alone for less than a minute. I glanced around the pod. A moment of rapture. This kind of planned catastrophic event sets the stage for the ultimate mindfulness. There was no past, no future. No goals, no regrets. No thoughts, no random rumblings of the mind. Only the Now. The Now was rich with gratefulness for a life fully lived. Yet it was not an emotion entrapped in thought. It was just there surrounding me. And I was not yet pumped with any narcotics!

The curtains moved, and in walked the nurse. "Time for something to make you feel good."

"All right! This almost makes it worth it!"

She clicked the little vial in place. Ahhhhhhhh. Ain't life good. Despite the promises by the anesthesiologist, though, I got cheated. The feel good juice lasted all of a few seconds, and then I was out cold.

Barry left to join Shea and await the arrival of the rest of the cheerleading squad. They gathered in the waiting lobby near the main hospital entrance amidst dozens of other anxious families. The group multiplied as the hours rolled by. First there were just Barry and Shea. Then Reva and Mickey with Mom in tow. Then Danny and Sharon, Barry's brother and his wife. Others came and went during the four-and-a-half-hour wait— Kathleen, Joe, Marilyn, Marshall, Rebecca, and Jim.

Several hours after the surgery had begun, Barry looked across the expansive waiting room as Dr. Thompson emerged from the hallway next to the elevators. His hair was hidden by his surgeon's cap, and his face mask was pulled down around his neck revealing a huge grin. As soon as he spotted Barry, he raised his hands and gave two thumbs up. Success! He rushed across the lobby and gave Barry a big, strong, congratulatory handshake to accompany his beaming grin. "We got it!"

Dr. Thompson was visually excited. Barry and Shea hugged as unobtrusively as they could. Everyone wanted to celebrate, but they were sensitive to the other tense dramas still underway in the neighboring huddles.

Dr. Thompson explained what happened. It was a difficult surgery, but he felt confident he had preserved my vision. He spoke of the challenge he'd encountered without revealing the scary details. I did not learn the full reason behind his animated spirits until two years later while doing the research for this chapter. The real drama was buried in my medical record.

> We used the Greenberg retractor system to elevate the frontal lobe. We removed spinal fluid, which allowed the brain to relax beautifully. [Is this a guy who likes his job or what? I want some credit, though, for relaxing my brain.] This gave us an excellent view of the optic nerve, and we could readily detect the tumor present as a vascular mass. . . .

> The tumor was very adherent to the optic nerve on the left. It also was dramatically compressing it, and the nerve was extremely distorted. I cannot emphasize enough how impressed we were about the degree of optic compression, particularly on the left. . . .

> The tumor also presented itself as a small knuckle in the opticocarotid cistern, further compressing the nerve. We worked to devascularize the tumor . . . depriving it of its blood supply. This softened it considerably and allowed us to debulk it internally. This then facilitated very gentle delivery of the tumor from the chiasm and nerve.

> There were small blood vessels that appeared to potentially be shared with the tumor, but these were carefully identified and cauterized using the highest degree of magnification. We removed the bulk of the tumor and then noted

that there was still a small component of it which was present beneath the nerve and potentially out into the optic canal from below the nerve. We worked very carefully, gently, and patiently in this region to completely deliver the tumor.

. . . we replated the bone, taking great care to provide a nice cosmetic coverage, especially at the region of the keyhole, where a separate small bur hole cover was fashioned to provide a nice contour.[I have nice contours now.]

What kind of person spends his days this way? Believe it or not, Dr. Thompson was a regular guy— "regular" in this case is a good thing. When I asked him later how he got into this business, he said during medical school he became fascinated with the brain and all the mysteries surrounding how it worked. Sounded reasonable. Indeed, I felt fortunate that his curiosity transformed into a Nashville-based passion. To this day, just a fleeting thought of Dr. Thompson makes me glow.

An hour after my skull had been pieced back together, I awoke in a recovery area. And I could see! At the end of my narrow bed sat a lone nurse at a table. A curtain surrounding both sides of the bed shielded me from the other recovering victims. Dr. Thompson had not misspoken in his prediction. He'd met the surgical challenge, and I "did great." It was a red letter day!

I was amazed at how alert I felt, a little woozy, but fully capable of conversation. I have no recollection of what I said, but I remember sitting up at a sixty-degree angle and talking with the nurse. I became a little nervous when she disappeared and was greatly relieved when she came back. Even in the postsurgical fog, I harbored a fear of being left alone in case I stroked out. I drifted off several times, and I was always comforted to see her at the end of the bed when I woke up.

Later I was moved to the neuro-Intensive Care Unit while they awaited the availability of a hospital room on the Neurosurgery floor. Reva, Mickey, Mom, Barry, Shea, Rebecca, and Marshall all came to visit in the ICU.

Balloons, flowers, Mom, Shea, and Barry were waiting when I arrived the next day in the unusually large corner room of the Neurosurgery floor. Friends and family came and went over the next couple of days. On day two after the surgery, my supervisor, Barbara, came by, and I was feeling well enough to volunteer suggestions about priorities at work.

After just three days, I was discharged. My alertness felt almost unnatural—are you supposed to feel this way after brain surgery? The most significant occupational challenge was getting a fork in my mouth. I had a locked jaw from a chewing muscle in the temple that had been cut for access to the skull. My mouth opened no more than an inch.

Some people would pay thousands of dollars for such a simple way to control weight. I got it free (sort of). I was discharged with a stack of Popsicle sticks, which I was to stick in between my teeth several times a day to gradually work my mouth open. I was told it might take a few weeks, but eventually I would be able to open my mouth wide again and shovel food in like everyone else.

Phase IV: The Aftermath

The day after I got home, Barry drove Shea to Atlanta for departure on a previously planned European tour with friends that we had not wanted her to cancel. Over the next few days, several folks waltzed in and out to serve as caretakers—Ava, Reva, Mom, Karen, the usual competent crew. Despite the fact that my skull had been drilled open, my brain jostled, my nerves frayed, and then my skull pieced back together with titanium plates and screws, I felt great. My vision was slightly altered. I had trouble seeing more than several lines on a page, but in a few months, my vision was better than ever. Maps became legible again, and my peripheral vision eventually returned.

I went back to work five weeks after the surgery and then retired two weeks later from a twenty-nine-year career in maternal and child health. Although I'd sailed through this latest, greatest ordeal with no surprises, I was in need of a long break. After nine major surgeries, substantial doses of radiation and chemotherapy, and the emotional ups and downs of cancerous and not-so-cancerous tumors, my body felt like a beloved, well-worn sweater that had been mended many times—still functional and a good fit, but fraying at the seams. Retreating to the rural woods of Nashville to write about my experiences seemed like the right direction for my tattered body and soul.

chapter seventeen

2006, JUNE

In June, 2006, one month after Surgery Number Nine, I woke up in the disintegrating body of an eighty-year-old with the gleeful presence of a four-year-old. The feather torture of herpes zoster (shingles) was tickling the unreachable underside of my skin covering the right side of my ribcage. The wide-band tourniquet created by my bodaciously firm mounds was constricting my chest. The right side of my face was still partially frozen in place, making the tiniest of smiles uncomfortable. The vacuum cleaner in my deaf ear was running at full volume. The peripheral vision in my left eye was snuffed out by an opaque cloud. And my body was anchored to the ground by a heavy fatigue.

Paradoxically, these lingering symptoms were nothing more than minor nuisances. They made me grateful to be alive, transporting me to that blissful place where I effortlessly embraced the moment. I had no debilitating pain, a freedom of mobility to walk, an above average capability to reason and talk (although I had recently introduced myself as Mary), and I had medical insurance.

I went for a walk down our driveway. The ragged old giant swallowtail butterfly flew by, the same one I saw each morning on my daily venture outdoors. I was able to spot her amidst all the other dozens of butterflies because she had lost over half of her right wing and a third of her left. Yet she still flew as smoothly as the day she'd emerged from her cocoon. I wondered if she felt as worn as she looked or if her search for nectar allowed her to maintain her focus, oblivious to her handicaps. As I watched her flitter around me, so close I could hear the faint whish, I thought, *I am a ragged old giant swallowtail. I still have color. I still flit.*

For the next few months, after departing from a professional career and full-time employment, I began flitting through my roles, from aspiring author, to caretaker of a feeble body, to rabid community activist.

2007

By 2007, I had stepped up to fill a leadership vacuum to help stop a massive commercial development from swallowing our pastoral community of Bell's Bend. My vision of a leisurely sabbatical was again interrupted. I had imagined rising without the aid of an alarm, meditating, dillydallying over a fried egg and fresh ground coffee, then adhering my buttocks to the chair in front of the computer to write about the tumor of the year. In the afternoon, I'd planned on strolling down the driveway to retrieve the mail and morning paper, then preparing a gourmet dinner of halibut with tomatillo sauce. Yet all these salivating expectations were replaced with increasingly stressful and chaotic days, phone calls, e-mails, presentations, and meetings. No one asked or expected me to serve as benevolent commandant to my neighbors. In fact, even Barry was unaware of the extent of my hijacked energy, time, and health. Yet my self-righteous passion for seeking justice and a spiritual fervor for our rural community sucked me in. It was a test of resistance, and I flunked.

I became a slave to the scattered agenda, gaining and then losing control of my healthy schedule on a daily basis. I accessed my management skills from my employment years to strategize and re-strategize about how to meet the simultaneous demands of my activist campaign, physical health, and state of mindfulness. As soon as I thought I had this unstructured, working-at-home thing figured out, a crisis would erupt with either my body or the body and soul of the neighborhood. I eventually set up shop for writing the book in Sandra's barn at the end of the driveway. Her husband and our good neighbor Charlie had passed away, leaving his tranquil law office in the barn unused.

The barn had no phone, no food, no pets, no e-mail. I walked or drove to the barn around 9:00 a.m. By around one o'clock, the hunger pangs would pull me back up the mile-long driveway, through the woods, and to my house for lunch. With the addictive joy of writing satisfied, I devoted the rest of the day to the Battle of Bells Bend, while also serving as VP of Internal Affairs for Barry's consulting business, having dinner with Mom, attending yoga class, and whatever I damn well pleased.

Later, with much of the book complete and several strategies underway for saving our community from urban sprawl, I set aside the final month of 2007 to devote solely to writing. For a Jew, December can be the most carefree month of the year. While most of the US populace becomes more and more frantic as the season of giving approaches the deadline of December 25, life for us eases to a snail's pace. Hence, December is the perfect time for a special project.

As I began to slide into my four-week retreat, giddy with expectations of hours of uninterrupted writing, a meteorite was hurled at me with a force I had not experienced in almost a decade – a mass of recalcitrant matter led by a band of viral aliens.

The jaw tumor, wedged in the right side of my throat for the past two years, had been a harbinger of trouble. All signs had pointed to a tumor of the timid, benign nature. This gal was a sluggish guest, content with snuggling up in the moist confines where the neck meets the back of the jaw. Technically, the tumor was called a schwannoma, emerging from the sheath of the sublingual nerve that controls the discharge of saliva and feeling of the tongue. Unlike her cancerous brethren, she showed no signs of interest in swallowing up her neighborhood. So we had decided to let her lie.

But in the fall of 2007, Ms. Schwannoma had begun to squirm, making the right edge of my tongue feel fat and ugly. Her link to my psyche created a periodic tingling sensation in both tongue and cheek, followed by numbness. I had been quite patient to let her reside indefinitely in my humble abode, but it was time to show her the door.

At the end of November, I presented my case to my neck tumor doctor, Dr. N., and his accompanying nurse and nurse practitioner. "This tumor has been in my jaw quite a while now. I'm wondering if it's time to take it out? I'm healthy and surgery-ready now. If we wait and the tumor grows, will the potential damage be greater as you attempt to separate it from the nerve?"

"There could be loss of the function of the taste buds. Maybe some numbness," he said.

"Well, if that's the case, the surgery shouldn't be a problem," I responded. "The taste buds on the right side of my tongue stopped functioning nine years ago after the acoustic neuroma surgery. And the right side of my tongue is already going numb from the jaw tumor. I don't even use that side of my tongue anymore. I'm less worried about the *current* risks of the surgery as opposed to the *later* risks of waiting."

Then I added, "One more thing. My COBRA insurance expires at the end of January. My new policy doesn't provide as much coverage, so if this surgery is postponed much longer, it could cost me thousands of extra dollars."

Much to my surprise, Dr. N. turned to his nurse and said, "Let's schedule the surgery for next Tuesday." He turned back to me. "I actually like doing this kind of surgery! Is next Tuesday okay with you?"

"Yes. I'm ready." I was elated.

Elation may seem like an odd reaction to news of impending surgery, but I had wanted to get rid of this gal for more than a year so I could lay to rest the persistent questions. Would it become cancerous? Would it grow, causing major nerve damage? Would it go through a growth spurt while I was down and out dealing with some other major onslaught? Surgery now was music to my ear.

"My husband leaves town on Tuesday afternoon," I said. "Is that a problem? How major is this surgery?"

"This is probably one-day surgery, not even requiring an overnight stay. As long as you have someone who can take you home, it shouldn't be a problem."

"All right then. Let's do it!" I gave a huge grin.

Dr. N. probably thought I was a medical masochist, and maybe he wondered if all of my nine previous surgeries had really been needed. I'm sure doctors run into all types of kooks, and I may well have been one of them.

I exchanged a warm, solid handshake with Dr. N. and thanked him for working me in on such short notice. Then I followed the nurse down the hall to schedule the surgery. About an hour later, I walked out with two appointments, a pre-operative appointment for the next day, and the surgery for 10:30 a.m. the following Tuesday.

After I relayed my plans to Barry when I got home, he said, "Are you sure you want to do this while I'm out of town?"

This experienced caretaker of Minda the Mangled Cancer Survivor smelled a rat. He wisely anticipated that no journey through the medical maze is without surprises, particularly when "they" have an opportunity to get a naked view of all the possibilities.

The next morning, I woke up with an air of excitement, as though I were hitting the road for vacation. The nagging little lady was moving out! Her irritating habit of tiptoeing around my house, bumping into the furniture, was coming to an end.

The Vanderbilt University Medical Center pre-op visit was the first demonstration of their commitment to outstanding patient care. After a brief introduction, the meek, but focused nurse practitioner moved right into the review of my medical history. She sat behind her desk with a laptop open wide, like a baby bird waiting for food. I sat comfortably on the other side of the desk ready to regurgitate.

She looked up from the laptop to make eye contact (ten points for good bedside behavior). "Wow. You have quite a history here. You've been through a lot. I want to make sure we get it straight, so let's go through this history starting with the first time you had cancer."

She devoted the next thirty minutes to unsticking the pages of my epic medical saga, showing a sincere interest in the physical fallout of these events. She was totally unaware this exchange was worth several hundred dollars of therapy, not to mention the value of accurately documenting the history for possible surgical implications.

Then she asked, "How are you doing *now*? Any problems?"

"I'm okay. Nothing major going on. I feel like I have some nondescript cold making me sluggish—you know—general malaise without any GI or respiratory involvement. Oh, and I also have this swollen lymph node on the left side of my neck." I turned my neck to the right to show her the protruding wonker.

This grape-sized nodule had startled me a couple of days earlier. As soon as I spotted it in the bathroom mirror, my fingers automatically went to the node, massaging it to detect size and soreness. Soreness usually meant an infection, not cancer. But this one was not sore. Not sore at all. Not good.

My first thought had been to press the panic button. Instead, I rationalized. Lately, I'd been feeling a tightness in my head that often preceded a cold. Though the sniffles, cough, and diarrhea had not surfaced, I decided that my body was harboring a virus.

That's it, I told myself. *I have a cowardly infection causing this node to swell up. No problem. Just ignore it, and it will go away.*

The nurse practitioner had already noticed the swollen node, and she had mistaken it for the tumor Dr. N. was going to remove, until I politely pointed out that this node was on the opposite side of my neck from the jaw tumor. She did not seem alarmed, and if she was not worried, I should not worry either, so I rationalized.

She said, "Let's do the examination, and I'll take a look."

I sat on the examining table while she performed the obligatory pre-op physical examination. After she listened to my heart and palpated the swelling in my neck, we both went back to our stations on either side of the desk.

"I think you need to go to Dr. N.'s office when you leave here and have him look at that node."

To avoid using up the rest of my day waiting to see Dr. N. while they tried to work me in to his busy schedule, I asked if she would please call his office. She did and his nurse said she thought he was aware of the swollen node and was not concerned. Still, she suggested that I mention it to him when I showed up on Tuesday for the surgery. She would talk to Dr. N. to make sure he agreed. Yippee. Back to the "forget about it" mode.

That evening I could not forget about it, so I showed the bulge to Kathleen. She looked worried and encouraged me to call Becca, Seth's nurse practitioner. That was not the response I was looking for, but wise advice nonetheless. When I called Becca later that evening, she urged me to come over for a face-to-face look, feel, and see. But rather than officially beginning the process of the Cancer Scare, I stalled. We settled on waiting for a couple of days to see if it would go down, and I promised to call her Sunday afternoon following the all-important Tennessee Titans football game.

I was a good girl and called Becca after the game, expecting her to participate fully in my plan to blow it off. When I told her it seemed to have shrunk a tad, she didn't bite. "You should still come over and let me feel it."

"I'm on my way."

A few minutes later I was sitting on the side of her bed while she palpated my neck. I could tell by the look on her face all was not right with my little bodily world.

"Since you're going to have surgery anyway on Tuesday, maybe Dr. N. can remove the node at the same time. My concerns are that it's not sore, it's pretty big, and there's just one swollen node on one side. With infection, we would expect to see more than one swollen node, and also it would usually be tender. I'll call Seth and see what he thinks."

She called him right then and there from the phone next to the bed. They chatted a few minutes, and then she hung up and gave me the verdict. "He's concerned, too. He suggests you call Dr. N.'s office first thing in the morning. Tell him Seth suggests he remove the node at the same time if possible." How's that for a taste of health care expediency when unencumbered by insurance hurdles?

Remove the node, sayeth Seth. With those words, my worry meter jumped up to Code Orange. The funk came hurling in from that hole in the sky and doused my body with one hundred extra pounds. I stayed cool, though. I showed minimal emotion. "Okay. I'll call his office tomorrow."

I stole a big hug from Becca and her husband and dear friend Joe, then walked out into the rain.

Other worrisome facts I had pushed aside were now swirling in the forefront of my mind, including a recent weight loss. On Friday during the pre-op exam, the nurse weighed me in at 118. I had not weighed under 120 pounds in almost ten years.

The next morning I called the nurse and left a message exactly as I was instructed. The nurse called back and left a message on my cell phone, but I didn't notice it until about two that afternoon when I was walking into a meeting with John, director of the Tennessee Environmental Council, to recruit support for our neighborhood battle against development.

The phone message was brief. "Dr. N. would like for you to come in this afternoon and let us biopsy the node. We'll be here until 4:30 and work you in."

I called her back as I stood in the parking lot outside the Council office. "Dr. N. says he would prefer to take some needle biopsies *today* and determine if the additional surgery is really necessary. He'll send the samples to the pathologist while you wait, so we'll know right away."

"Thank you. I'm heading into a meeting, but I'll be there by four o'clock."

By the time I hung up, I was shaking. I thought, *In a couple of hours I will know if I have cancer again.* My gut told me all of this was for naught. I have an infection. But guts don't have brain matter, so what do they know? I felt doubt, because I couldn't ignore the disturbing signs: loss of weight, no tenderness in the node, a lone mass on one side, and the worried looks on the faces of Kathleen, Becca, and the pre-op nurse practitioner.

I gathered myself and my worried psyche together and walked into John's office. While we were talking, my eyes began to water, and my voice began to shake. Then my emotions burst forth in a free-for-all.

"I'm . . . sorry . . . John . . . for dumping on you . . . right now." *Gather thyself. Breathe. Release. Sighhhhh.* "I just found out I may have lymphoma again. I don't really think I do, but I'm scared. I just got a call from the doctor's office, and they want me to come by this afternoon for a biopsy."

John responded in a most sensitive way (for a guy). "Let's hold hands and pray. Dear God, may our dear friend Minda find grace and mercy. Please keep her healthy. In Jesus' name. Amen."

Then, with a tender sensibility, he asked, "Was it okay to mention Jesus? I didn't mean to offend you."

"Absolutely no problem. It was from the heart. And I truly appreciate you taking the moment to offer a prayer. I think I'm okay, for now anyway, so let's talk business."

An hour later, as I drove to Vanderbilt, I turned on the local sports radio station for a diversion. Titans talk. How calming. In the lobby of Dr. N.'s office, as soon as I settled into a chair for the nerve-racking wait, I called Kathleen. Her office was in the same tower, so she offered to come up and help diffuse the flutters. Within five minutes, she walked through the waiting room doors toward me. Love is more calming than Titans talk.

A few minutes later Kathleen and I were escorted into an examining room, and Dr. N. was soon at my side. "Let's see what we have here." He palpated my neck. "Yes, that's a pretty big lymph node. How long have you had it?"

"It actually popped up a few days ago."

Dr. N. glared a few seconds at my neck and then gave me his expert surgical opinion. "Removing this node is not as easy as it looks. It is next to your carotid artery, and I may have to tug on some nerves to get it out. I'd also like to avoid having to cut you on both sides if it's not absolutely necessary. So let's do a needle biopsy now. We can send it down to the lab while you wait. There's no need to take it out if it's infectious. How does that sound?"

"Sounds like a good game plan to me. I'd rather not have any additional surgery if I can avoid it. Besides, I really think it's nothing, and the sooner we confirm that, the better."

Dr. N. departed. A few minutes later, in came the surgical pathologist followed by a resident and a medical student. They reminded me of a youthful Mother Goose trailed by two goslings. Their combined age could not have added up to a hundred years.

I was not a novice to the pleasures of a needle biopsy of a growth in the neck. The procedure sounds and looks archaic and painful, but it is relatively innocuous. My fear stemmed mostly from the outcome, not the procedure.

"I've seen you before," I told the pathologist. "You performed a needle biopsy on my neck last year." At the time, she'd been the resident gosling getting practice.

After we'd adjusted my position on the table, I said, "I'd like to make a special request. Would you please clean the site really well? Last time, I got a staph infection. I was pretty miserable, actually."

I wanted to tell her, *Last time you probably didn't clean the site well enough, so when you inserted the needle, you injected me with the staph sitting on my skin. Do you know how easily preventable that is?*

Of course, I didn't say all that. Instead, I held back my lingering disapproval and remained as cordial as a hostess at a tea party.

The resident turned my head to the side, exposing the protruding node. "Is your head comfortable?"

"Yes. I hate to be a pest, but please wipe the spot well."

The resident tore open the package of alcohol-soaked gauze and wiped my neck. Kathleen came over and held my hand. They did not give any anesthesia for this easily accessible node, either topical or injected, so when the needle pricked my neck, it must have looked barbaric to Kathleen, who was more squeamish than I was at this point.

"You will feel some pressure," said the resident. "Here we go." She slid the needle slowly into the lymph node and aspirated. Nothing. The first sample was dry.

"Let's try again. Patients tell us it looks worse than it feels," Mother Goose told the resident and student. "Is that true?"

"Yes, it's true. It really isn't bad at all." I was *not* just trying to set the needle pusher at ease. It was the truth.

This time she hit the mark and got some tissue. "Let's get two more samples," she said. "Here we go again. You'll feel some pressure." She got what she wanted with stick number two.

"One more time, and we'll be done."

In went the needle. Pressure. Slight discomfort.

"Done!" exclaimed Mother Goose. "Good job."

She turned to face me and said, "We're going to take this down to the lab right now. We should have a report within thirty minutes."

In walked Dr. N. "Okay now. You can stay, or you can go home, and I'll call you when I get the report."

I turned to Kathleen. "Do you mind sitting here with me?"

"Not at all."

"We'll just wait here if that's okay with you."

"I'll be right across the hall if you need anything," he replied and walked out.

Kathleen and I were alone. She looked at me, rolled her eyes, and then we both smiled at each other, though mine was more of a Batman Joker smile with a slight upward curve at the corners. Our ironic smiles mirrored our sentiments: *Here we go again.*

Kathleen and I tried to keep some banter rolling as we waited. It worked. In no time, Dr. N. was back.

"I just got the report. They could not say it was cancerous, but they could not say it was *not* cancerous."

"You mean the sample was not good enough to make a conclusion?" I asked.

Dr. N. turned to Kathleen. "She knows too much." He turned to me. "So I think we should go ahead and take it out, because we don't want to make you worry for a while and then have to come back in a month and undergo another surgery."

"I guess this means I can stay overnight, right?" One-day surgery was not my cup of tea. If I had to be slashed, I wanted to have ready access to more potent drugs and a hospital bed with numerous positions for comforting a bruised body.

"Yes," he said. "We can arrange that. I'm sorry we don't have more definitive news, but we'll get to the bottom of this tomorrow. I'll see you in the morning!" He gave me a hug and walked out.

Kathleen and I walked together to the elevators outside the clinic lobby. I was more shaken than ever. I had expected to receive conclusive confirmation of my rationalizing. Instead, the door toward another confrontation with the cancer demons opened wider. I yearned to believe the inconclusive results were the result of a set of crummy samples. I was having difficulty mustering up a plausible self-sermon, though, to bolster my wilting confidence.

Before Kathleen and I parted ways, she gave me one of her powerful looks of love and a big hug, and said, "I'll come to your room as soon as I can after the surgery. I love you."

"I love you, too," I told her, trying to maintain my composure. What started out to be a straightforward one-day surgery on a benign tumor had suddenly become a potential nightmare. "Thanks so much for coming over. I really thought this was going to be no big deal."

I started to get teary-eyed and felt the need for personal space. "I'll see you tomorrow. . ." My voice trailed off, half question mark, half period. Kathleen got on the elevator, while I stayed behind to cry.

I gave myself a couple of minutes to wail in a corner of the hallway by the elevator. Fortunately, no one came along to invade the much-needed privacy.

After I spilled the tears and moans, I pulled my cell phone out to speed-dial Barry.

"Hey. I've got sort of good news and sort of not so good news." I told him about the inconclusive biopsy. "Damn. This really sucks. This was not supposed to be about looking for cancer."

"Well, the good news—and it really is good news— is that it's NOT definitely cancer. Let's focus on that for now," he said.

"You're right. That *is* good news. And this surgery is going to be much easier than the last two surgeries. All right then. I'll see you at home." His wise words lifted my spirits.

I will not belabor the gruesome details of this, the tenth surgical tale I've shared with you. The short version is that I was in the hospital one day and night. Barry left for the airport after I was wheeled away to the OR, but he received a call just prior to boarding the plane that the surgery was over and all was okay. Ava stepped in to coddle the patient through the night—a good thing because this not-so-major surgery led to a rumble-tumble evening as the pain meds were unable to contain my body's discontent.

Shea had been quite nervous about this surgery. This was the first time she had not been by my side. She was now a young woman adjusting to life in New York City as an assistant fashion designer. During her twenty-two years, she had witnessed far too many assaults against her mother. Some had been pretty hard hitting, so it was a challenge for her to think positively before the surgery, particularly from a distance. We talked the evening after the surgery, but my shaky voice did not comfort her. I called her the next afternoon so she could hear a stronger voice.

"Hi, sweetie. How are you?"

Shea said, "I'm doing much better than yesterday, which was terrible. Right now I'm walking down Houston Street, and it's starting to snow."

"Oh, Shea. I'm so glad today is better. Snow is wonderful—it's like sunshine!"

Shea paused a moment, then said, "Mom, *you* are my sunshine."

In that moment, I felt like the most fortunate woman on the planet.

A week later, I received The Call. Neither the tumor nor the node was cancerous, so in the cosmic scheme of things, I was flying high. Down on earth in the land of the healing, however, I was stumbling around in a fog.

For several weeks, I was jarred awake each morning by my neck's paradoxical resistance to both movement *and* stillness. I endured stretched nerves, confused muscles, a re-paralyzed face, and a rampant virus that had taken control of my body, none of which was expected. Upon rising and swinging my legs out of bed, I became cognizant of the jelly-like matter in my head that had once been a functioning brain. I felt like a robot with someone else at the controls. And that someone else had dialed my speed to the lowest setting.

Three weeks after the supposedly minor surgery, while I was still in the fog, Barry and I flew to New York City to help Shea get settled in her new apartment. As I struggled up and down the six floors to and from her no-elevator apartment in the Lower East side, I suspected something was amiss. My body's ability to snap back from surgery had always instilled me with pride, but this time around was different. Was it a new anesthesia? Advancing age? The stress of the David vs. Goliath battle to save our rural neighborhood? I pushed my way through the family holiday, convincing myself I just needed more time to heal.

As the weeks and months unfolded, my face, neck, shoulder and accompanying nerves and muscles gradually started working again as a team, and the thick fog in my head slowly began to recede. I was slowly piecing myself back together, hoping soon to ready to resume an active life. But I was in for another rude awakening. It was not meant to be.

chapter eighteen

> More and more I have come to admire
> resilience.
> Not the simple resistance of a pillow,
> whose foam returns over and
> over to the same shape, but the sinuous
> tenacity of a tree: finding the
> light newly blocked on one side,
> it turns in another.
> A blind intelligence, true.
> But out of such persistence arose turtles,
> rivers, mitochondria, figs—
> all this resinous, unretractable earth.

> "Optimism" by Jane Hirshfield,
> from *Given Sugar, Given Salt*.
> © Harper Collins, 2002.

2009

Each of us has one role that defines us more than anything else—parent, nurse, painter, nurturer. I am a survivor of health challenges. I'm either on my way up or on my way down. The direction I'm headed and my stamina, or lack thereof, define what is left of me. When I am on the rebound feeling robust, I am an activist. Without the stamina, I just am. Between the *I* and *am* lies both a very long and a very short space. Few things are sustainable in this exhausting space. Writing is. This book has enabled me to describe the many ups and downs with my body and the challenges of getting back on my feet.

After the neck surgery, I set off on a whole new journey. I was and still am both on my way up and on my way down. You would assume traveling in two directions at the same time means I'm making no progress. Quite the contrary, this awkward state of being has pushed me into places both physically and spiritually far beyond anything I have previously experienced.

The most recent leg of my journey began with a new diagnosis, Epstein-Barr virus-related B-cell lymphoproliferative disease. That's a fancy name for a tug-of-war for control of my white blood cells, or lymphocytes. On one end are millions of healthy B-cell lymphocytes fighting infection and cancer. On the other end is a virus named after two Jewish dudes – Epstein and Barr.

This stealthy virus hunkers down in the heart of the B-cells, causing debilitating fatigue and abnormal cell proliferation. The most lethal manifestations of the infected B-cells are deadly mutations that multiply until a nasty lymphoma cancer develops. The end product is destruction of the mothership (me)—and ironically the virus, too.

Seth explained our mission: to contain the insidious Epstein-Barr virus (EBV). An uncontrolled virus could launch a life-threatening cycle. If EBV-infected B-cells became cancerous, they would multiply and create more homes for the virus, which would stimulate even more cancer cells.

The Epstein-Barr Virus—Lymphoma Cycle

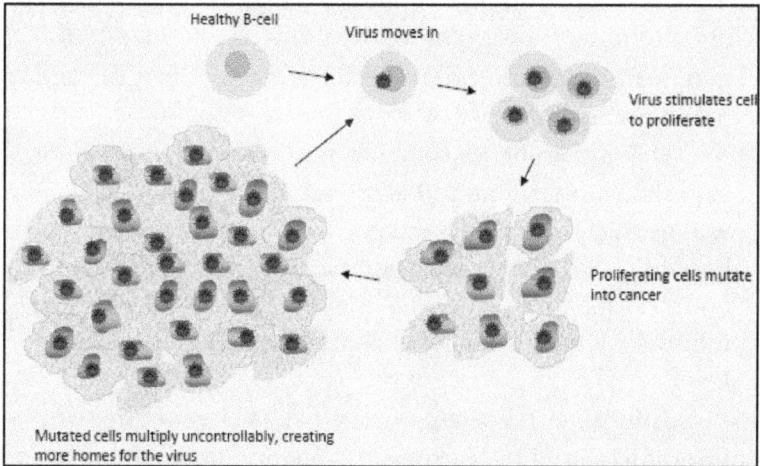

How do you stop this evil tyrant from taking over? Unfortunately, the wizards have no answer this time. The proliferation of the Epstein-Barr virus in my lymphocytes has created a catch-22. Launch an attack to stall the growth of the virus, and we may create a more vulnerable environment that will spur the growth of cancerous lymphoma cells. Treat the condition like a full-blown case of cancer, and we may ultimately weaken the host (me) and my natural immune system so the virus gathers steam.

The best we can tell, I'm about a 7.5 out of 10 on the continuum, with my lymphocytes revealing *features of polymorphic B-cell lymphoma*. With the rise and fall of the EBV, as measured in a periodic blood sample, my energy wobbles back and forth from fair to pitiful. On days when the virus seems to be taking a nap, I leap into productivity, writing for a few hours and then making calls to raise money or organize a public hearing. An antiviral drug, the only innocuous treatment offered, has not worked. So I've constructed an alternative program of healing—daily meditation and reading of the Sh'ma, acupuncture, T'ai Chi, and pomegranate juice.

The recommendation for now from my team of experts is no treatment. Let's wait and watch. Maybe it will go away. Maybe it will get worse. I awake each day hopeful I will have the stamina to function for a few hours. Amazingly, I'm feeling better than I have in months, with the virus at a mighty active, but stable level.

This potent Epstein-Barr virus is demanding and unpredictable. I'm learning the enemy, and the enemy is learning me. We'll come to a truce soon. And in that truce may be an enduring peace.

NOW WHAT?

Some time has passed, and despite the tenacious assault of the Epstein-Barr virus, I have finished the book. Further, we won round one of derailing the $4 billion development that would have devastated our rural neighborhood in Bell's Bend. I also learned double—no triple—no exponentially more—lessons about living in the moment, responding to daily demands of life, holding true to who you are, and staying alive and healthy (mostly). This book is about the latter, so let's get down to the tricks of the trade for steering your way through the ever changing world of health, wellness and not so wellness, as seen through the eyes of a thirty-eight-plus-year cancer survivor.

MINDA'S FIVE STAGES OF RESPONSE TO CATASTROPHIC DISEASE

My health odyssey has taken me down two parallel paths: the physical path with its twists and turns through the maze of the health care system, and the spiritual path with a more linear journey. The first path has left my physical package bruised and battered and sometimes fearful of the battles yet to come. Fortunately, the almost four decades on this arduous path have led to considerable success at actively navigating the five stages of response after a diagnosis.

Stage 1: Panic—Holy Shit!

Minda freaks out, cries a lot, is short-tempered, and needs a lot of love.

Stage 2: Manic Willy-Nilly Research

Minda goes online, calls doctor and nurse friends, combs the shelves of Whole Foods for the Magic Potion, and jumps at any and all of the nine-hundred-ninety-nine suggestions made by well-meaning friends and relatives.

Stage 3: Focused Research

Minda calms down, reflects on what she's learned so far, and then identifies what questions need to be answered and where she is going to obtain the answers to get through the medical maze with minimal damage. With answers in hand, Minda develops a well-thought-out game plan.

Stage 4: Action

Minda is knowledgeable, confident, and ready to leap into action to find that special place where contemporary medicine meets alternative care— surgery, chemo, or wait-and-watch, along with meditation, prayer, and yoga. She's ready to roll.

Stage 5: Acceptance

Minda has found peace, knowing the outcome will be what it will be.

I've not been a quick learner. On the other hand, having passed through these stages many times, I now can sense when I am transitioning from one step to the next, an awareness helpful in and of itself. Moving through these stages, I've observed both subtle and blatantly obvious dos and don'ts and, bit by bit, I've evolved an unwritten guide. This guide has helped me rack up the wins in this game and still be here to tell my story.

I've been a bit reticent to share these lessons. They are based on my own personal experiences and temperament. Therefore, they may or may not work for others. I describe them here hoping some useful nuggets are transferable to others' medical challenges. These lessons are a blend of old age, middle age, and New Age wisdom, and I imagine their usefulness will depend the urgency of the trauma, patience, persistence, and luck.

MINDA'S TOP SEVEN LESSONS LEARNED FOR NAVIGATING OUR HEALTH CARE SYSTEM

Lesson One: *Know Thy Body*

Feeling good leads to feeling better. Feeling lousy leads to feeling lousier. As we age, the gap between good and lousy widens. To prevent falling into the gap and never emerging again, we must learn to listen to our bodies. Our bodies usually are good communicators, giving all kinds of signals, like the far-off whistle of an oncoming train. If you are listening, you can hear the train coming long before the railroad crossing lights begin to flash. The earlier we catch both the bold and the subtle cries for help, the sooner we will be back out of the gap and into the full light of wellness. In the case of cancer, listening well and acting early may mean the difference between life and death.

Sometimes our bodies can be passive-aggressive communicators, though, with vague signs further muddled by mixed messages. How can we straddle that line between wise caution and paranoia?

First, take advantage of the millions of public and private dollars America has invested in early detection. Cholesterol checks, Pap smears, breast self-exams, mammograms, PSA tests, colonoscopies—do them. Don't delay. Did you know that, if caught early, more than ninety percent of cancers can be treated successfully? Listen to the wisdom of Dave Barry:

> Mr. or Mrs. or Miss or Ms. Over-50-And-Hasn't-Had-a-Colonoscopy. Here's the deal: You either have colorectal cancer, or you don't. If you do, a colonoscopy will enable doctors to find it and do something about it. And if you don't have cancer, believe me, it's very reassuring to know you don't. There is no sane reason for you not to have it done.

> Dave Barry.
> From the McClatchy Newspapers
> *The Miami Herald*,
> One Herald Plaza, Miami, FL 33132

Second, know your family history so you can be screened for your own additional risks. If your mother had diabetes, be screened and stay on the lookout for the signs of this disease. It will be much easier, less traumatic, and less costly to treat if caught early.

Third, know how your machine looks, feels, and sounds when it is running smoothly and treated well. For example, do you exercise regularly enough to know your body's potential for robust health? What does the rhythm of a healthy heartbeat feel like when you are sitting, taking a leisurely walk, or climbing stairs? Is your stamina usually charged enough so by workday's end you have plenty of energy to fix dinner, or do you feel a need to hit the sack as soon as you get home? Is that lump in your breast a life-long resident, or has it just appeared? Has a mammogram or professional examination confirmed the lump is not worrisome?

Finally, become familiar with the internal workings of your worry meter. Worrying for a while is okay. "For a while" wears out its welcome, however, when it puts a significant dent in your quality of life. Do you wake up in the middle of the night, unable to go back to sleep? Can you no longer concentrate long enough to make it through an entire page of this book without your mind wandering to your latest ailment? Have you spent the past six months blowing off that pain in the right side of your belly, but it is now on your mind most minutes of every day? You may be better off solving the mystery with a trip to the doctor.

I admit on more than one occasion I have snubbed my body's cues, turning a deaf ear to her increasingly loud pleas for help. In 1997, when my acoustic neuroma was just taking root, my eyelid starting twitching incessantly. This seemingly harmless symptom was followed by a loss of balance at dusk. Then the phantom saliva sensation in the corner of my mouth became more persistent. But I was not paying attention. I even ignored the worried advice from a well-respected neurologist, Robbie, my brother-in-law. Just one of the numerous symptoms might not have cracked the barrier of denial, but the combination should have broken through. As I ignored them for more than a year, the tumor probably grew from a vulnerable seedling to a well-anchored bush.

Lesson Two: *Choose Thy Doctors as Thou Chooses Thy Car*

When you know something's up, it's time to shift from your rationalizing delay tactics to a consult with an expert. Sifting through the choices of health care providers requires shopping around with the same passion and attention you would for a new car. Would you choose a make and model without checking out the stats on its mileage, reliability, or safety? Would you buy a car sight unseen? Your car will be ready for the dump long before the driver expires, so doesn't the driver's body deserve the best mechanic you can find?

A relationship with a doctor is like a marriage—it may last a lifetime, with the doctor standing by your side for better or worse. Or the doctor may be with you for a just short period, more like a one-night stand that meets some desperate need. Either way, you want the right partner. And unlike most marriages, you will want and need many partners. So how do you find the right candidate best matched for you and your current ailment?

Seek out referrals for the type of doctor you need from friends, relatives, colleagues, and especially nurses and other health care providers who work in the specific field of medicine. The most knowledgeable opinions based on firsthand experience often come from non-MD health care providers, for instance, as a physical therapist or a nurse. These professionals hear directly from the patients and observe firsthand the strengths and deficits of the doctors in their field. If you reach a dead end, ask folks to call folks they know who may have firsthand experience or knowledge.

I have learned the hard way that doctors can be the least informed about the shortcomings of their colleagues. Undoubtedly, it is natural to hesitate to criticize friends or colleagues. One doctor is unlikely to say of another doctor, "I heard Dr. X. was negligent . . ."

On the rare occasions when doctors query their patients about the adequacies of their referrals, the patients may not be forthcoming because they don't want to offend their doctors. And doctors can be the last to learn when a physician with a twenty-five-year, distinguished reputation starts dropping the ball because he's lost his passion for the work. So how can we expect the doctor to learn about the true quality of care provided by his colleagues if he, his colleagues, and his patients are self-censored?

Surgeons are the exception to this rule. Asking surgeons or anesthesiologists *who have observed your candidate in the OR* is a surefire way to tap into a firsthand, graphic testimony. The surgical colleagues often will reveal their opinion by the inflection in their voice. "He's fabulous! An amazing surgeon. No question about it. I would recommend him for any member of my family!" Bingo—you've probably found your man.

"He's a good man. He does good work," delivered with minimal emotion means you should probably find someone else if you can.

Unfortunately, you or someone you know cannot always talk directly with a surgical colleague, anesthesiologist, or anesthetist who has worked with the said candidate, in which case you will have to rely on your interview with the surgeon (see questions below). Three additional caveats to contemplate when choosing a surgeon are:

1. The most desirable traits in a surgeon are excellent technical skills, not bedside manner. And don't fall into the trap of assuming a

surgeon *must* be top-notch if he practices at a famous academic research hospital. Despite popular belief, the hospital should be secondary to the doc himself.

2.   Of course, direct testimonials from patients are important, too. But beware of opinions from a cousin or friend. They usually have observed only one set of experiences, while nurses and physical therapists have observed many. The individual patient's perspective may be valid, but soliciting more than one point of view is a wise, cautious approach.

3.   Once you've narrowed down the choices to one or more candidates, schedule a consult or exam to interview each one. Come prepared with several well-thought-out, open-ended questions that will fill in the gaps of your confidence in this candidate. Open-ended questions require a descriptive response beyond one or two words like yes or no. Be prepared with your list in hand. Time will go by fast, and you'll want to make good use of it. Remember, the doctor is there to help, but others are waiting.

I've offered a few ideas here, although it's best to adapt them or think of your own, depending on your most urgent needs. For example, are you looking for an expert surgeon for a one-time event, or a long-term relationship with a primary provider? Remember, despite what your mother might have believed, physicians are not gods, and rarely, if ever, are they good at everything.

It's prudent to prioritize and direct your questions toward your most pressing needs. A physician confident in his skills and knowledge will gladly answer your questions and will look forward to working with you if you're actively sharing the responsibility for your health. Also, consider taking someone with you, in case you feel too intimidated or stressed to ask the questions and hear all the answers. Examples of questions to ask are as follows:

1. "I'm trying to learn as much as I can about my condition. Would you please help me understand and visualize what specifically is going wrong?"

2. "I'm not quite following you." (This question gives the doctor another chance if she has gotten too technical or not detailed enough.)

3. "What is different about my case that might present a challenge?" (This question addresses the doctor's expertise in dealing with *your* situation.)

4. "This next question is a little awkward to ask, but it's important for me to be as confident as possible in your experience. How many patients a week do you see (or operate on) with my problem? For how many of these cases are you the *primary* physician/ surgeon?" (Someone else in the practice may be the lead provider for patients with your particular situation.)

5. Prior to a physical examination, ask, "What are you looking for?" (This question often yields many pertinent facts not yet discussed.)

6.   "My plan all along has been to get two opinions. It's not personal. I'm just trying to get as much information as I can so I can be as confident about the procedure as possible. If you (or your spouse) were having this procedure done, who would you go to for a second opinion?" (A good doctor will not be bothered by this request.)

By the time you've gotten answers to your questions, you should have a general sense of whether you've found a keeper. Remember, your first attempts may be brief since most of us feel uncomfortable with this type of probing.

If a doctor appears agitated or frustrated with your questions, you can acknowledged his discomfort in this way. "I realize I have a lot of questions. I hope you'll be patient with me as I try to understand what's going on." However, if after several attempts, the doctor still avoids answering, does not explain things in terms you can understand, or does not provide answers specific to your situation, this is a tell-tale sign that you should keep looking.

One more point to consider about the Big Search for Mr. Right. If you have a rare or puzzling condition and cannot find an adequate candidate in your community, look elsewhere, even outside your state. Insurance should cover the cost, except maybe the travel expenses, which are tax deductible. Most likely you'll have to jump through several hoops to get approval, but it can be done. Few conditions out there have not grabbed the curiosity and passion of at least one devoted physician somewhere in the country.

With a rare condition, you want to take the time to find that person whose life's purpose is to decode the medical mystery brewing in your body. Go online, focusing on sites affiliated with academic research centers. In the end, a scientist or specialized facility may have the best shot at solving the mystery. Thorough research will save you a lot of time, money, and frustration—and maybe your life. In the worst-case scenario when no specific diagnosis or treatment is identified, your research will still most likely yield more knowledge, so you'll feel less fearful of the unknown and more at peace with your condition.

Once you've closed in on the best doctor you can find with the time, resources, and patience you have, keep your eyes and ears open during each visit. You deserve a compassionate and attentive quality of care. If you have not landed the right provider, move on. Acknowledging you've chosen the wrong person is tough, but the sooner you break the tie, the sooner you will get the care you need. Don't forget, you are paying for this service.

Lesson Three: *Understand the Condition Thy Condition Is In*

You may already know the fundamentals about your condition, but unfortunately, these basics will probably not be enough to guide you through the snarly concourse of decision making. What else do you need to know, and where will you find this information? Doing the necessary research may become like a second job, yet it may be one of the most important jobs you'll ever have. Your performance may affect who and what you will be for the rest of your life—in both good and not so good ways.

I've found six key questions which are essential to answer at this point in the medical journey. Your main objective is to understand enough about the problem so you can actively discuss your options and also communicate when an important detail or symptom has been overlooked. With this information in hand, you also will be better able to sort out the many well-intended suggestions from friends and family. Getting answers to the following six questions has been as important to my long-term survival as choosing the right doctor.

1.   What are the complete medical names and other descriptors used to label your specific diagnosis? What do these terms tell you about the nature of the beast? Where is it? How aggressive is it? For example: there are many types of breast cancer, but only one is called invasive lobular carcinoma with focal ductal features.

2.   Can you visualize which parts of your body are in trouble, where they are, and who else resides in the neighborhood? The latter is important to better understand the potential side effects of the disease or treatment. Elementary cartoonish images of your body parts may be sufficient, as long as they help you visualize and comprehend. For example: a two-centimeter mass in the glands of the breast where milk is made and stored with no evidence of disease in the ducts or neighboring lymph nodes.

3. With a physical image in mind, what is working or not working that is causing the problem? For example: cells in the lobules of the breast whose sole purpose is to make milk are multiplying out of control (with no baby in sight).

4. What are the top two or three treatments recommended? How does each solve the problem? How do the treatments differ? For example: lumpectomy with radiation versus a modified mastectomy.

5. What are the potential problems or risks with each treatment? For example: lumpectomy with radiation may lead to possible lifelong risk and fear of recurrence, whereas mastectomy may lead to possible sexual and self-esteem issues.

6. What are the risks of just waiting and watching?

To avoid spending endless days trying to find this information in terms you can easily decipher without a medical dictionary by your side, consider the following steps:

1. Ask your doctor these questions in a face-to-face visit, and then ask her or her nurse for a pamphlet or brochure. If she does not have information on hand, ask where you can obtain written information. The more patients who ask, the more likely the practice will keep this information on hand.

2. Seek a second opinion if you have a serious condition. You will be amazed at what you will learn from having two different people explain your condition to you. The two explanations are often as revealing as getting directions to a house in the country from two different people. One will fill in the gaps for the other or alert you to a piece of the puzzle you misunderstood.

3. Go online. Choose Web sites ending in .edu (universities), or .org (nonprofit such as Mayo Medical Clinic or American Cancer Society) or .gov (government agency such as National Cancer Institute). Avoid sites ending with .com or .net (for profit). Be attentive when sites are sponsored by laypeople vs. professionals. Both can be useful, but it's important to know the difference.

4. Once you've obtained answers to the questions, you may want to review what you've learned with your doctor and nurse and ask them to clarify or correct your findings if you've misunderstood or omitted an important detail. It's hard not to feel shy or embarrassed about an elementary level of knowledge, but try to remember most health care providers will be pleased you are taking such an active role in your care.

Lesson Four: *Defend Thyself—Learn the Art of Self-Advocacy*

Becoming an effective patient is like any other endeavor. You get out of it what you put into it. And it takes practice. Practice and experience yield success. Success yields confidence. Confidence yields motivation to keep practicing, to keep self-advocating.

You are the one and only CEO of your ever-evolving personal health care team. Each of your physicians is one of many advisors on the team—some with long-term tenures and leadership roles, others with short stints. Punting this responsibility entirely to your doctor can be a big mistake.

Physicians often operate from a two-dimensional vantage point. Their perspective on any diagnosis, prognosis, or mode of treatment is based primarily on scientific evidence and their experience in their own practice. One or both of these sources can give doctors unwavering faith in their recommendations. They rarely give as much weight to your individual situation simply because there is no literature on you alone, with your specific history and genetics, nor will there ever be. So it's a gambling game.

With ample scientific evidence in the literature and "proof" from other patients, the odds are the doctor will be on target or at least reasonably close. Sometimes, however, a doctor's previous knowledge and experience will cloud her vision instead of aid it, so she will miss the elephant in the room. *You* will sense the big, smelly elephant, though, and should not ignore it. Often, if you're persistent, something magical happens. The doctor's eyes are opened, and the next time around, she will see, hear, and smell that anomalous elephant.

I have witnessed many times and in numerous settings the significance of doing your own research, engaging in an honest dialogue with your physician, and together weighing the pros and cons of the options. You may not always agree with your doctor, and a gut reaction may not bring clarity on which route to take, but in the long haul, these conversations will lead to better decisions, better health, and greater peace of mind.

By contrast, anger, resentment, and guilt are common reactions to poor medical decisions. Yet most catastrophically wrong choices are avoidable. In addition to honest dialogue about the treatment choices, four additional cardinal rules should dramatically reduce your odds of a bad decision:

1.   Ask to see all pathology and radiology reports.
2.   Get a second and sometimes a third opinion for invasive treatments.
3.   Read drug inserts.
4.   Do not allow thy insurance provider to masquerade as thy doctor.

Doctors are being pressured to see more and more patients in less and less time. And so it follows, they may quickly scan the *pathology or radiology report*, reading only the summary or perusing for key words. In addition, not all doctors will interpret findings in the same way. Obtaining a copy of the report allows you to read it yourself and then, if necessary, to pass it on to another doctor for a second opinion. You will also have a copy for your files in case other related conditions occur in the future. Twice I have had physicians with excellent reputations overlook a new tumor on an MRI even though it was cited in the radiology report. By the time one mass was acknowledged, it had grown fifty percent.

In another instance, a prestigious physician failed to report a diagnosis cited in CAPITAL LETTERS in the summary at the top of the pathology report *and* mentioned in the narrative description eight times, with a cautionary note indicating the worrisome nature of the findings. My unsophisticated level of knowledge with the terminology did not impede my ability to detect the ominous words and numbers the doctor had not disclosed to me.

Invasive procedures are invasive, which according to Mr. Webster means, "intrusion by an attacking army." Invading the human body comes with risks and consequences. Most of the time when invasive procedures are recommended, the benefits outweigh the risks, for example, a mastectomy for breast cancer. However, in some instances, a wait-and-see or another noninvasive approach may be sufficient. If the procedure is significantly invasive to you (it is a personal decision to judge just how much invasion you can tolerate), then take the time to seek a second opinion.

Drug inserts are long and unwieldy. Reading a drug insert can bring on a big, bad case of paranoia. Will I have diarrhea, itching, suicidal tendencies, or worse yet, a heart attack from swallowing this innocent-looking tablet? Yet one question merits wading through the gobbledy-gook: *Is this drug recommended for my situation?*

On occasion, for valid reasons, doctors choose to prescribe a medication approved for conditions other than yours. Sometimes, it's related a related condition. Other times, serendipitous use of the medication has shown benefits for other ailments, but the studies have not yet made their way through the rigorous Food and Drug Administration approval process. Either way, you deserve an explanation from your doctor. You may want to choose a more tried-and-true method, or you may agree with your doctor's advice. Bottom line— your choice should be an *informed* choice.

When I had a small squamous cell skin cancer on my face, I read the insert for a topical medication my doctor had prescribed. This type of skin cancer was not insidious, but potentially more risky than basal cell cancer because it could metastasize if left untreated. My eyes floated across the side effects and chemical structure and eventually landed on the approved uses. Squamous cell cancer was not on the list.

When I asked the doctor about it, he claimed the med *was* approved for squamous cell cancer. This situation was probably not a big deal, but with my history, it made me feel a little worried. So I scheduled a consult with another dermatologist who gave me another side of the story. He informed me the drug had not been shown to be effective with squamous cell skin cancer. He also said he was unaware of any topical treatment used without surgery for this type of skin cancer. I stopped using the cream, and he surgically removed the tissue. I left his office with a zero on my worry meter. In the end, it might not have made any difference, but it was my choice, not the doctor's, to determine the risk I was willing to take.

There are times when playing nice with the *insurance company* just doesn't stop the bleeding. And when you don't feel well, the last thing you want to do is to yell into the phone at an innocent health insurance employee about the need for more bandages. But be prepared to do it. Ask for the manager. Demand the manager's manager. If you have dutifully paid your monthly premiums for health insurance, and the procedure is not an explicit *noncovered* expense in your policy, you have a right to appeal a decision. If you don't ask, you don't receive.

The doctor is your first line of defense with the insurance company. Sometimes, a simple order from your doctor will do the trick. For example, most insurance companies usually approve only one night in the hospital for a modified mastectomy without reconstruction. Don't let the insurance company scare you. You are having major surgery. If you want to get home to your own bed as soon as possible—no problem. However, if you want to remain in the hospital with all the comforts—adjustable bed, pain pump, round-the-clock care—just ask your surgeon.

For more complicated snags, your doctor may need to make a formal written request for approval of the procedure she is recommending. If there is no affirmative response, you may need to jump in. Patience is helpful on the first, second, and perhaps even the third attempt. If patience doesn't work, try anger and tears. You'll know when it's time to give up. But at least try. Self-advocating for treatment integral to my healing not only resulted in an extra night in the hospital, but also led to coverage in another state for rehabilitation therapy not available in Tennessee.

Come hell or high water, more change is a-comin' in our health care system. The change will not be flawless, and it is unlikely to be massive enough to fill

in all the holes. We shouldn't expect it to be. A health
care system that meets all our needs all the time is too
costly. And too flexible of a health care system will be
unmanageable. Learning the art of self-advocating for
the best care at the right time by the most appropriate
provider is a skill you will always need, regardless of
the size or shape of our health care system.

Lesson Five: *Heal Thyself*

It is easy to feel lost, hopeless, and confused when
under attack from forces seemingly beyond your
control. The medical treatment itself can push you out
of the picture as an active player in your healing
process. You begin to feel like a bystander at a wrestling
match with no control over the outcome.

The quickest way out of this conundrum is an
activity that enables you to feel you are spinning *into*
control rather than *out of* control. Swim, walk, garden,
meditate, paint, knit, play music, eat massive quantities
of veggies, imagine, laugh, cry, and/or pray. Do
something—anything—to feel that you *are* a player in
your body's healing.

It is up to you to find what works best. Does
gardening calm your agitated soul for at least the hour
your hands are in the dirt? Does a brisk, daily walk
through the park energize you? Does a good night's
sleep help you wake up with a refreshing sense of
hope? Do the concentration and harmonics of playing a
guitar allow you to lose yourself in the music? Do two
glasses of pomegranate juice a day help you feel you're
blocking the cancer from moving on to other cells? Does
a daily practice of mental imagery allow you to feel
you're oiling the cogwheels of your immune system?

Does a daily prayer help you quiet your fears of the future?

At first, the impact of these activities may be temporary, breaking the downward spiral of despair for just a few moments. With regular practice, the moments turn to minutes, the minutes to hours, until eventually the periodic fix rests lightly on your shoulders throughout the day. And you'll know where to find an extra dose when you need it.

With this go-to activity, you will no longer feel like an outsider in your own body. A lightness, more frequent smiles, and even acceptance will replace the tense shoulders, the dreary fog, and that unhealthy feeling of helplessness. Whether the activity itself truly contributes to your healing is secondary to the improvement it makes in your attitude. Chances are, once your attitude has changed, the activity *will* heal and will also invigorate your role as a valuable partner in the healing process.

After my tenth surgery, the complications overwhelmed me. I knew I needed to do something, but I was so fatigued and frustrated with my condition that I couldn't beg, borrow, or steal from all the lessons of the past. I finally followed up on a recommendation made months earlier by Seth as well as by Julie, my yoga and T'ai Chi teacher. I made an appointment with Susan, a physical therapist specializing in an esoteric method of therapy called myofascial release.

I walked into her office at 2:00 in the afternoon. At 3:30, I walked out with a new lease on life. After months of depleted physical and psychological stamina, I found the yellow brick road. The primary effect of Susan's therapy lasted only a couple of days, but it tapped into a wellspring of hope and energy to create my self-structured, self-healing program. It was work, mind you, but I found a way to reconnect with the helpful, rather than helpless, person inside me. Then I became a real partner to the rest of my health care team.

During this time of floundering after Surgery Number Ten, as well as after other surgeries, I had to make several attempts to regain that sense of control. These trials brought blips of relief, but nothing stuck long enough to garner the staying power I needed. With each surgery, I learned (or relearned—I'm a slow learner) it's very difficult to recover if you can't take time to focus on healing. *You've got to clear the decks to make room to heal thyself.*

This concept is probably one of the most difficult aspects of re-attaining your well-being. We have a very difficult time letting go of our many commitments— work, family, community service, play. But until we let go of all but the bare essentials, we miss the best paths back to a sense of control and wholeness.

Americans resemble alcoholics when it comes to saying no to numerous commitments throughout the day. Most of us have to hit rock bottom, such as feeling our life is threatened, before we can utter *no* repeatedly. While you are in the throes of a life-altering trauma, you have a great excuse to just say no. No one will doubt your good judgment to put your health at the top of the list.

Simplify your life by stopping to examine the debris scattered about on your decks, and toss overboard everything but the bare essentials. By this, I mean *minimum* work and family commitments— nothing else. This will free up the time, energy, and psyche to see your most helpful priorities in a new light.

Think about this. With each of the priorities on your schedule, will it matter five, ten, or fifty years from now if you were there? Think back over the last year to meetings, parties, phone calls, or community obligations. Could they have survived without you? Would you have survived? Would missing an event have significantly altered your life?

Remember, your changed priorities are probably for a limited period of time. And they are crucial to your journey toward well-being. (Please note I have not used the term *wellness* here. In some instances, the wisest goal for the present is to just find peace with your newly tempered state of health, which may or may not be defined as *well*.)

Take advantage of offers for help from friends and family. They have their own need to give and will appreciate your forthright requests. There is a time and place for giving, and this may be your time for receiving. When friends ask how they can help, tell the truth and give specific examples. "Clean my house. Bring over a meal, but PLEASE, no more vegetable soup, in fact steak would be nice...and don't forget the beer and M&Ms for Barry. Send thoughtful cards instead of energy-zapping emails, visits or calls. Take me to the doctor. And most importantly, send oodles of love and prayers in whatever faith, form or fashion feels right."

Once you have cleared the decks, you will be astonished at the sigh of relief from deep within. You now have plenty of elbow room to determine your next step, uncluttered by a racing mind or body hurrying off to the next destination.

When you feel well-oriented to the spaciousness, be prudent and pace yourself. Gradually add one healing activity at a time until you've constructed a practicable program to get you mentally, emotionally, physically and spiritually back on your feet. Several trials and errors after my last surgery, I finally settled on a forty-five-minute daily regimen of deep breathing and meditation followed by a reading of the Sh'ma prayer and a self-Breema treatment, a gentle stretch and touch to help bring my body and mind into balance.

Once you've done the hardest part—cleared the decks and constructed a plan—it's time to reorient yourself to make sure your health is your top priority. Is your plan for well-being at the top of each day's agenda? Not second, not third, or not "if I have time." But the *top* priority for each and every day?

Finally, practice your program daily, or five days a week at minimum. It won't work if you just think about doing it. Practice makes perfect—or makes you moderately less imperfect.

Lesson Six: *Find Thy Balance Between Taking Control and Letting Go*

Beginning in my late teens, I worked for years on gaining control over the health of my body. Eating wholesomely, practicing yoga and meditation, living in the country, growing my own food, baking my own bread, hiking, minimizing stress, and avoiding guilt. My motivation to do more, control more, was fueled by my success. When Round Two of Hodgkin's laid me low, more success from these efforts fueled my motivation and pumped up my ego. I felt like I was pretty damn good at this stuff. I was Woman. I could survive. I was in control.

Then I got breast cancer. Boy, was I caught off guard. It shattered my confidence. Suddenly I felt angry and betrayed by my will to be healthy, and I was catapulted back into the realm of helplessness, ready to let the doctors have at me, come what it may.

Prior to the breast cancer diagnosis, I had unknowingly set myself up for a fall. In my mind, I believed that I had created an impervious armor to protect me from future assaults. My perception of the forces controlling my health was somewhere in the neighborhood of eighty-five percent Minda, fifteen percent Other. This was my error.

As I groped my way through breast cancer, I began to accept the limitations of my control, and surprisingly, this freed me from guilt that I had not tried hard enough. Since that time, I have spent years running back and forth between grasping for control and letting go, searching for the elusive balance.

I've become more observant of where I am in this search. When I ignore my self-healing tactics and let go completely, I feel a heavy dose of guilt from not doing enough. On the other hand, the pressure of trying to assume too much control leads to an overbearing fear of failure that has no off switch.

Where am I now? Right in the middle—where equal doses of taking control and letting go balance each other. Pretty stable territory. No guilt. Minimized fear. Maximum peace with what I can and cannot do.

I've been here before, but eventually, I wander off in one direction or the other. I'm guessing I will be here a while—longer than ever before, though not forever.

Because the seventh and final lesson has been beaten into Patient 2410 too many times to ignore:

Lesson Seven: *Thy Learning Never Ends*

These seven lessons are the compilation of hard knocks received on the long and bumpy path of my health. On October 16, 2009, I was diagnosed with Epstein-Barr-related diffuse large B-cell lymphoma, Stage IV. I completed six rounds of chemotherapy, and as I write this, I am in remission. Forty years have passed since I arrived at St. Jude with my first bout of cancer. I'm no longer an active St. Jude patient, but I am and always will be Patient 2410.

Chances are, the rest of my path that lies ahead will be riddled with more challenging obstacles. The massive exposure to carcinogenic radiation and chemotherapy has combined forces with my body's genetically rooted lust for growing tumors—I'm a sitting duck. I am forced to acknowledge I may very well not be around next year.

I've not yet done a stellar job of accepting this knowledge. Living in the moment lifts my mood, but the effect is brief because capturing the mindful moment takes hard work. It's similar to navigating a narrow bike lane separated from the busy traffic by only a thin white line. Just one small distraction—a pothole, a barking dog, a passing car radio—can take you across the line into a collision.

Since I was fifteen years old, I have tried to follow this difficult path to mindfulness, one tiny step at a time. This path parallels the ups and downs of my health path, and in many ways, it has been more difficult, yet much more rewarding. It is the path to spiritual grounding, a path you want to stay on as long and as often as you can.

Along this path, magical windows open to reveal the healing truths that coexist with pain, sorrow, and confusion. Regardless of where you are in your health or search for help, a view through these windows leads to a simple peace—a place where you can feel sorrow and joy at the same time. A place where you exist only in the moment, no longer fearful of yesterday's brain tumor or tomorrow's biopsy. These views are so beautiful, so calming, you begin to feel the physical abuse that brought you here is a small price to pay.

By traveling these two parallel paths for almost four decades, I think I ought to have seen it all by now. Yet new windows are still opening up with wider views. I keep learning that there is always more to discover about dodging the unforeseen and seemingly endless barrage of bullets.

The bullets keep coming. . . .

I keep living. . . .

I keep learning.

epilogue

On the evening of October 6, 2011, Minda Lazarov, my mother, was at home alone enjoying the peace and serenity of our house deep in the woods of Tennessee. As often happened, she was tired, feeling a little sick. She was in remission from her fifth round of cancer, but the Epstein Barr Virus still had its tight grip on her body, and her heart was worn out from repeated rounds of radiation. Every now and again she would send out warning signals, saying, "You know my heart is only working at forty percent. It could give out any day now."

I would respond with typical daughterly angst. "Oh Mom, please. Can we not talk about that! I'm planning on you being here forever."

That evening, she spoke to all of us by phone—my dad, my grandma and me. After dinner, she cleaned up the kitchen, put a Dr. Pepper in the freezer for an ice cream float and pulled out a can of pineapple juice to add to the half empty orange juice jug (one of our favorite Minda tricks). Her heart must have skipped a beat, a feeling she experienced from time to time in her weakened state. She grabbed for the counter, slamming the pineapple juice against the sink.

As her heart took its final beats, she sat the can down, squatted to the ground, and lay back in the middle of the kitchen floor—the same kitchen where she'd spent years cooking, mothering, hosting, enjoying. And then, it seems, her heart stopped. Our dog, Skylar, nudged her arm, asking her to wake up, but she didn't respond. So there they lay through the night until my dad arrived home from a business trip the next afternoon.

When my dad spoke the words, "Minda is dead," I felt a sense of relief. I know that seems odd, but I had been fearing my mother's death for as long as I can remember. Earlier, my parents and I had met with our rabbi, post-diagnosis, to talk about what we were feeling. I didn't say much. Nor did my dad. My mom said she was at peace with the idea of dying. She had fought and won enough battles, and if this last one took her, then it was her time. Her energy to be the brave warrior at battle after battle had waned.

But I was mad at her. How could she be content with leaving? I needed her. I needed her to want to stay with me. What I didn't know was that the opportunity to discuss life and death, and most importantly, her being at peace with her own death, would guide me through my life after her passing.

As much as I missed my mom and felt sad for my own loss, I was happy for her—happy that she went in peace, with no pain, in her favorite place. In my warped mind, I thought I would melt away as soon as my mother passed on. Instead, I found that she still lives within me and in so many other people.

I am a bit biased, but from what I can tell, the wisdom she gained through the five cancer demons, two brain tumors and ten major surgeries rubbed off on more people than I will ever know. The luckiest part of it all for me is that she wrote down her thoughts. This has been her journey, and maybe some of her words of wisdom will rub off on you, too.

Shea Lazarov Sulkin, Daughter of Patient 2410
September 30, 2012

If you feel inspired, please make a donation to St. Jude Children's Research Hospital, 501 St. Jude Place, Memphis, TN 38105, or at www.stjude.org/donatenow.